beginner's guide to
power
walking

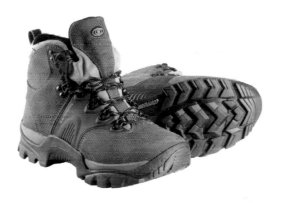

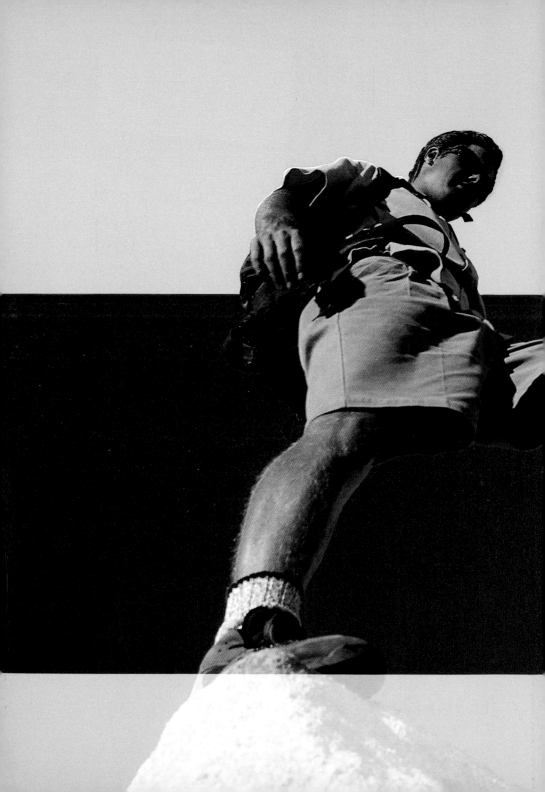

beginner's guide to
power
walking

JANICE MEAKIN

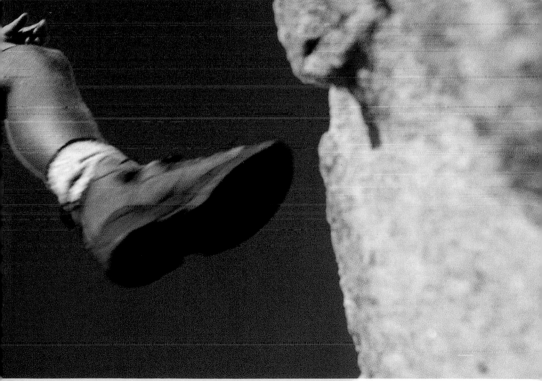

BARRON'S

First edition for the United States,
its territories and dependencies, and
Canada published in 2003
by Barron's Educational Series, Inc.

Conceived and created by
Axis Publishing Limited
8c Accommodation Road
London NW11 8ED
www.axispublishing.co.uk

Creative Director: Siân Keogh
Managing Editor: Brian Burns
Design: Axis Design Editions
Editors: Emma Clegg and Conor Kilgallon
Production Manager: Sue Bayliss
Production Controller: Juliet Brown
Photographer: Simon Punter

All inquiries should be addressed to:
Barron's Educational Series, Inc.
250 Wireless Boulevard
Hauppauge, New York 11788
http://www.barronseduc.com

Library of Congress Catalog Card No:
2002107468

ISBN 0–7641–2432–3

NOTE
The opinions and advice expressed in this
book are intended as a guide only. The
publisher, author, and consultants accept
no responsibility for any injury or loss
sustained as a result of using this book.

Printed and bound by Star Standard Pte
Ltd, Singapore

9 8 7 6 5 4 3 2 1

contents

beginner's guide to power **walking**

foreword

Power walking is the easiest, safest, and quickest way for most people to get fit, stay fit, lose weight, and experience the physical and psychological benefits of regular aerobic exercise.

In an age when increasing numbers of people are overweight, underexercised, and overstressed, power walking puts the zip back in your step and makes you feel on top of the world. We both lived very busy lives 13 years ago. Unfit and overweight, we tried jogging, exercise bikes, and all the exercise fads going, until we discovered the benefits of power walking. Power walkers walk tall, and they are leaner, more energetic, less stressed, and more motivated. And motivation is where it all begins.

The *Beginner's Guide to Power Walking* is the smart way to get started and gradually build up toward a power-walking pace. The guide is split into six motivational plans. Whether your goal is to improve fitness, maintain fitness, or even train for a walking marathon, the training schedules and regular self-assessment stages ensure that you begin and progress safely and effectively at the level most suitable for you.

Essential guidelines for avoiding injury are provided, with information on warming up and cooling down and suitable stretches for working the muscles used in walking. Statistics show that the dropout rate for people taking up exercise can be as high as 50 percent, often due to injury and pushing at too high a level to begin with. Because almost everyone walks, walkers start out at a comfort level, gradually increasing their pace without straining their bodies.

As well as the core training program, the *Beginner's Guide to Power Walking* includes advice on the full range of walking accessories—the way to choose suitable walking shoes and information on equipment such as pedometers, heart-rate monitors, and the clothing needed for walking in all types of weather.

Nutritional guidelines are provided in the healthy eating section, and tips on how to prepare for a marathon are also included. The *Beginner's Guide to Power Walking* is the complete self-coaching source for all exercise walkers.

MAGGIE HUMPHREYS & LES SNOWDON

AUTHORS OF *The Walking Diet*, *Walk Aerobics*, and *Step It Out*

why power walk?

A book about walking? We were designed to walk, so surely it must be simple. Well, yes, you learned how to put one foot in front of the other as a toddler and it is not a skill that is ever forgotten. But if the thought of walking up a hill or walking more than a mile makes you feel breathless, then you may not have experienced the joy of a long walk in the countryside, the easiest form of exercise in the world, or that wonderful feeling of achieving a goal for which you have trained and prepared hard.

So how does power walking differ from ordinary walking? The activity of walking may seem fairly straightforward —you pick up each foot and put it down again, don't you? Years of walking may make you think that you are already an expert, but if you were to pick up the pace, walking for a

power walking gives you all these added benefits:

peace
Fresh air, pleasant scenery, and a chance to watch the world go by alone or with friends—you are at peace with your thoughts and with the world.

energy powerhouse
Any brisk activity improves the efficiency of your metabolism, stops you from feeling lethargic, and inspires you to do more with your time. Once you get that buzz, you will laugh at that old excuse that you didn't have enough time or energy to exercise.

health gains
Once you take this first step to improved health, you will notice that other parts of your lifestyle have changed for the better. Your quality of sleep will improve, you may favor healthier foods, and smoking and heavy drinking will be less appealing. You may also lose the aches and stiffness that you thought were just the normal signs of aging.

health insurance
Regular walking stimulates your immune system, uses calories, and improves circulation. As a regular walker, you will also have less risk of diabetes, heart disease, and some cancers. We are all living longer, but it is established that active octogenarians have less disease, more independence, and better mental health too.

weight control and improved body form
Walking burns calories just as surely as any other brisk activity: you use 100 calories for every mile you walk, whether it takes you 12 or 20 minutes. You will notice the difference in your shape too: your legs and buttocks will tone up, especially if you have been using hilly routes.

self-confidence
Fitness makes you feel good about yourself, proving that you can achieve a goal that you have set yourself. The motivation and sense of achievement that you gain can spill over into all areas of your life, improving your career and relationships, too.

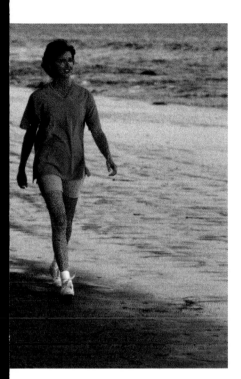

of injury. It also carries many of the health-giving aspects of an aerobic activity such as running or cycling— a good workout for the heart and lungs and the production of feel-good hormones. In fact, walking has so many benefits that it could be called "today's best buy in health." Some enlightened doctors prescribe a walk instead of a pill to treat depression. Any activity that uses calories burns sugar and fat, and helps you to keep to a healthy weight, which can prevent diabetes and heart disease. Power walking strengthens your whole body and helps you to make the transition from a leisurely walk to a speedy pace.

The best thing about walking is that you can do it absolutely anywhere, and for a short walk you don't even need to change your clothes. Always have comfortable shoes handy, however, so you can give your feet the support they need whenever an opportunity to walk arises.

walking success stories

1 Dave Couper, self-employed management consultant, 57

Dave was an enthusiastic runner who used power walking after a hip replacement to regain his fitness. He was surprised to find that he got a "walker's high" that was equivalent to the feeling he got when running. What's more, using hills, intervals, and "sprints" in his training had the same effects on his heart rate and state of mind as running, but without the strain on his joints.

2 Alyson Davies, housewife and part-time teacher, 39

Alyson was physically fit before she married. After having three children, she began to experience back pain, and running, in her efforts to get fit, made it worse. When a friend suggested she could use walking to manage her back pain and return to her former fitness, she rose to the challenge with enthusiasm. Some nine months later, she walked the Race for Life (a 26-mile [42-km] Cancer Research UK event) in 7 hours and 22 minutes.

whole day or carrying a heavy load, you would soon find that posture and technique, not to mention comfort and fitness, make a big difference in how easy it is. That is where power walking comes into its own—a sport for fitness and for pleasure, which involves using schedules and techniques to help you get the most power out of your body when you walk.

the benefits of power walking
Power walking gives you all the benefits of general walking— low-impact exercise with a low risk

getting started

With all those benefits just waiting outside the door, you are probably already planning your first walking route. However, before you hunt out those old shoes, there are a few more things you should know to make your walks safe and comfortable. This introductory section addresses any concerns you may have and explains how to make the most of the training schedules later on.

using this book

In the first chapter, you will find all you need to know about choosing shoes, clothing, essential accessories (and not-so-essential ones) as well as some dietary tips and advice on maintaining your energy levels. This is followed by a look at walking technique in terms of warming up, cooling down, and stretching as well as advice on dealing with injuries and keeping your motivation high.

If you already walk for an average of 30 minutes a day and want to know how you can increase your pace,

Your current level of walking fitness will help you to choose your starting level (see pp. 46–47).

progress to longer walks, or train for an endurance event such as a weeklong trek or a marathon, then note the different levels and goals listed in the second chapter on training schedules. These can be followed exactly or modified if you find you are fitter than you thought or you have a period of inactivity that sets you back a week or two. The schedules can keep you going when your motivation lags and help you achieve your goal in the shortest time without risking injury.

On the other hand, although all walks are good, you may slip into a comfortable routine that doesn't stretch you enough, in which case your body needs a combination of strengthening and stamina workouts to go faster and farther. Read through the safety checks on pp. 12–13 before you start, and then dip in and out of the sections as required. The final chapter looks at long-term goals such as how to train for a marathon and how to keep your weight down by walking regularly.

1 complete beginner	**2** starter level	**3** refresher level
if you can walk for 5 minutes comfortably.	leisure walker who is already walking at a moderate pace for at least 30 minutes a day.	if you have had a break in your program or you can walk for 45 minutes at a brisk pace 3 days a week.

excuses, excuses

"I'm too busy for long walks"

Take every opportunity for walking, even if it is only a 5-minute trip. Once walking becomes a habit, you will find that you are getting fitter and reaping the benefits and you may then enjoy the prospect of longer walks. But you don't have to train for the marathon—if you want a specific goal, aim for the shorter distances or the "holiday trek."

"Even ordinary walking makes me feel breathless"

Although breathing harder than usual during activity is normal, severe breathlessness is usually associated with a lack of fitness. Regular short walks will achieve the desired fitness level sooner than you think. Start at beginner level, and don't increase the pace until you feel comfortable. However, if you are still becoming breathless with gentle increases after a couple of weeks, consult your doctor.

"I feel silly"

One of the best reasons for using walking to get fitter is that you don't even have to look as though you are exercising. When you first start, you don't need to exaggerate your arm movements. If you look around, you will see that people all walk at different paces, so you'll just be one of the quicker ones.

"I can't walk fast enough"

Power walking is a technique rather than a pace. It involves using your arms more and only walking faster as you get fitter. You can walk at whatever speed you like, but you should feel comfortable and relaxed. Technique, terrain, fitness, and leg length influence pace during power walking, although long legs don't necessarily mean a faster pace.

"I have medical problems"

Walking is the best sort of exercise for most medical conditions: it is even used in supervised rehabilitation after very serious problems, such as heart attacks. Unless you have real problems with mobility, then you can walk at your chosen pace. Even if you have no medical problems, talk to your medical advisor before increasing your activity level or taking up a new activity.

the sing, gasp, talk test

Use this test while you are walking: if you have enough breath to sing, then you could work harder; if you are gasping for breath, then you need to slow down. The ideal scenario is to be breathing faster than normal, while being able to talk at the same time.

4 **intermediate level**
if you are a regular walker who walks for 1 hour at a brisk pace 5 days a week.

5 **upper level**
if you are an experienced walker or trekker who walks every day for 1 hour at 4 mph (6.5 km/h).

6 **advanced level**
if you are a walker who spends at least 1 day a week walking for 2 hours and 1 hour every other day walking at $3^1/_2$–4 mph (5.5–6.5 km/h).

one step at a time

Avid walkers have to start somewhere—and it is normally just outside their front door. Setting off on the wrong foot, as the phrase goes, can actually set you back and stop you from achieving your goal. So follow the principles on these pages and you can look forward to years of enjoyable and satisfying walking.

how fit are you?

Finding out how fit you are is the first step to achieving whatever goal you have set for yourself. If you are thinking of going somewhere, you plan your journey from where you are starting and not from where you would like to be. Four out of five people who aren't active enough to benefit their health think that they are fit. It is all too easy to overestimate your fitness

and start at a level that you will find too hard. Avoid this by starting at the complete beginner level if you haven't been regularly active for over a year.

But before you think about improving your fitness, what is your state of health? Answer the questions in the health checklist opposite and if you answer "yes" to any of the questions, then see your medical advisor before you begin training.

fitness check

How far can you walk at a brisk pace without getting out of breath?

- If you can't walk for 15 minutes comfortably, start at the complete beginner level.
- If you can walk for more than 15 minutes, measure out a mile (in the car) and see how long it takes you to

five steps to SMART goals

have a Specific goal

Choose a target or timed distance, for example 1 mile (1.5 km) in 15 minutes; 1 hour of continuous walking; one of the goals in the training schedules; or a weight loss of 10 lb (4.5 kg). Write it down and keep it where you will see it every day (such as on the refrigerator door).

how Measurable is it?

You can check that you are on target by splitting up the ultimate goal into weeks or months: follow the schedules to stay on track. If your aim is to lose weight, only weigh yourself once a week.

Is your goal Achievable?

Always be realistic with your goals. Training for a marathon in 8 weeks would be unattainable if you have only just started.

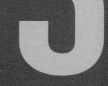

walk the distance. If it takes more than 20 minutes, start at the complete beginner level. If it takes less than 20 minutes, start at level 2.

■ If you want to start at the complete beginner level but find that it is too easy, then work through the first few weeks more quickly.

■ If you haven't been active for the last five years or are 40-plus years old, then take the first few weeks gently.

anywhere and everywhere

If you walk whenever you can, you can easily increase your daily walking time by 30 minutes—a great start to establishing a regular pattern of walking. Walk up escalators and stairs, walk to the store, walk to and from work, and walk to friends' houses. If you must take the car, park it farther away from your destination than you might otherwise have done.

walk with friends

Have a chat walking with friends or take their dog for a walk with you. Or get some friends to share your walking goal, or part of it, and join you on the longer walks. You could also join a walking group or, if you can't find one, start your own.

HEALTH CHECK

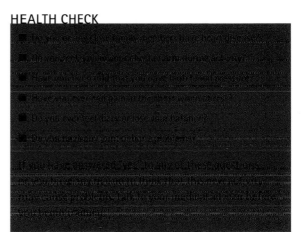

be Realistic

If time, mobility restrictions, or any other barrier prevents you from building up your walking distances, then you need to modify your goal to one that is within your capabilities.

set a Time deadline

If the date of your goal is too vague or in the distant future, it is easy to find excuses to put off training or even starting at all. A goal 3 to 6 months away is ideal—enough time to train but not too far away. If your ultimate goal needs to be reached for a vacation next year, then also set a realistic goal for halfway through the year.

pitfalls to avoid:

• agreeing to someone else's goal when you are not really convinced that it is the right one for you

• sticking rigidly to a goal that has become impossible because of changes in your life or health

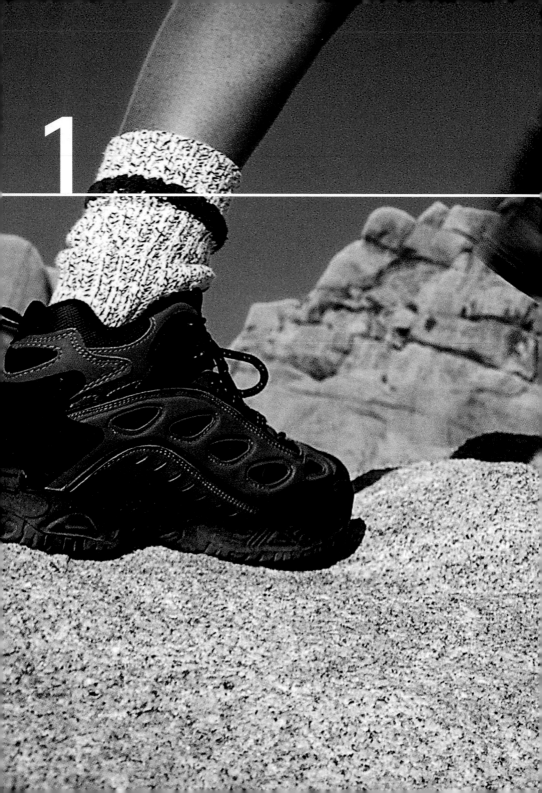

booted up

Getting the most out of walking is easy once you know how. Beginners don't have to do it alone: this chapter tells you about the equipment and accessories that you need for training as well as for participating in the event. No special gear is required for short walks, but specialized shoes and clothes, and a walking kit can make all the difference in the world to your comfort and will keep you safe during the training schedules, as well as encourage you to keep going. This is followed by dietary advice and an outline of walking techniques—warming up, maintaining correct posture and technique, and treating injuries.

walking in step

Choosing the right footwear for the type of walking you plan to do is the most important part of your preparation. You may need more than one type if you want to walk on different surfaces, but keep in mind that ending up with the wrong footwear can be an expensive mistake. A pair of walking boots costs as much as a pair of trainers and you may only wear them once a year if most of your walking is on roads or sidewalks. The advice on the next four pages will help you to make the right choice the first time.

if the shoe fits

A well-fitting shoe is probably more important than the cost. Always try new shoes on in the afternoon when your feet are warm and at their biggest. Take with you the type of socks that you intend to wear and remember that for hiking boots to be comfortable, you will also need hiking socks. There are almost as many specialized socks as shoes nowadays, and a specialized retailer can advise you on the assets of each type.

Because your feet flatten and push forward when you walk faster, hiking boots and trainers often need to be at least one size larger than the shoes you normally wear, and there should be at least a thumb's width (your own, not the assistant's) between your big toe and the end of the shoe. Your foot should feel supported, but not restricted, and your heel should not move up and down in the shoe as you walk.

shoes for all occasions

Whether you buy sandals, walking shoes, hiking boots, or trainers, certain rules apply to all types of shoes (see pp. 18-19 for shoes for different terrains). Your shoe should have support to prevent your foot from rolling excessively inward (overpronation) or outward (supination). This support is called stability, and how much you need depends on your biomechanics (how your feet and legs move as you take each step). A shoe should also provide cushioning to protect your joints and muscles from jarring. A store with expert staff can assess the way you walk or use computerized technology to measure your gait as you walk before recommending suitable shoes.

fit and feel

There are many specialized shoe manufacturers, from Reebok to Hi-Tec, each with their own unique qualities. Although the scientific-sounding names may make you think that you should choose one over another, the fit and feel is more important. Some shoes are simply too narrow or too broad, so don't be sold a product on a piece of indispensable technology at the expense of the shape of your feet. Try on a range of brands, and choose a pair that feels comfortable in the store—if they aren't comfortable there and then, they certainly won't be when you get home. If you find you have made the wrong choice, most retailers will exchange them as long as you have not worn them outside and you return them within a reasonable time limit.

have my shoes lost it?

It is difficult to gauge how long a pair of shoes or boots should last because it depends on the mileage, your weight and gait, and the hardness of the terrain. The lower your mileage and weight and the softer the terrain, then the longer they will last. Generally, because you can't always judge that a shoe has outlived its usefulness from the outside, you should replace your training shoes every 350–400 miles (563–644 km) or every year, whichever is soonest. If you find a pair of shoes that fits well, buy two pairs so that you don't have to break in a new pair just before the day or week of an event. If you start to experience knee pain for no apparent reason and your shoes are more than six months old, you may have walked more miles than you realize, so change them first, before you undertake expensive treatment.

four steps to finding the right shoe

1 Use specialized stores—supermarkets are not the place to buy shoes for serious walking. The expertise you need to make the right choice is only available at outdoor, walking, and sports retailers.

2 Avoid general shoes—these may be cheaper and they may appeal to your eye. They will not, however, have the features that you need to support and cushion you through miles of walking.

3 Assess the merits of designer trainers—at the other end of the scale, expensive shoes are not necessarily better than cheaper ones. Find out what you need first, in terms of stability and cushioning, and then find out what they cost.

4 Consider a shoe's weight—this can vary enormously and lighter shoes may not offer the support you need. Hiking boots are heavier than walking shoes, and trainers can feel extremely light by comparison. Be guided by what you need for the terrain, and by your own weight and motion control, rather than what the shoe feels like in your hands—after all, it is your feet that will be wearing them.

walking on air

It is possible to walk in any type of sensible shoe, but the shoes you choose should allow you to achieve your goal in maximum comfort and also suit the terrain and distances you intend to walk. Shoes for walking fall into four main categories: hiking boots for uneven and rocky ground; walking shoes for long distances on trails or uneven terrain, trainers (cross or trail trainers) for walking on roads or sidewalks, and trekking sandals for summer walking on rocks and trails. If you only want to buy one type of shoe, decide on the most versatile type to suit a range of terrains and elements—walking shoes or cross trainers may fit the bill. If you have weak ankles, hiking boots will offer the extra support you need. A sturdy pair of waterproof hiking boots will probably cost more than other types of shoe, but never use cost as an indication of suitability: walking on roads or sidewalks can be uncomfortable in shoes designed for rigid support.

shoe care

A pair of shoes can last for a long time if they are well cared for. After each walk, brush off any dry mud on the uppers. Wash or brush them with a hard brush if the mud is wet, and let them dry out naturally away from direct heat or sunlight. Protective oils or material-specific creams will prolong the life of the uppers and stop them from becoming hard and rigid.

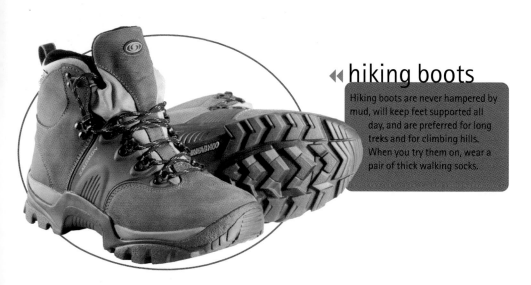

◂◂hiking boots

Hiking boots are never hampered by mud, will keep feet supported all day, and are preferred for long treks and for climbing hills. When you try them on, wear a pair of thick walking socks.

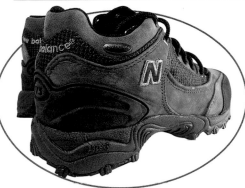

walking shoes

For all weathers and most terrains, walking shoes are the most versatile shoes for walking. They are, however, less suitable for hard, even ground because they provide less cushioning than trainers.

cross trainers ▶▶

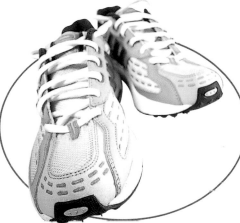

Cross trainers are probably the most widely available and popular shoes. Different types of trainers can also correct supination (leaning outward), overpronation (rolling inward), and provide extra cushioning. A specialist store can tell you the shoe that will suit you best.

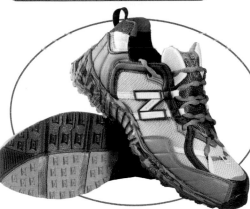

◀◀ trail trainers

Trail trainers offer better grip on muddy ground, but other types of shoe are more versatile.

sandals ▶▶

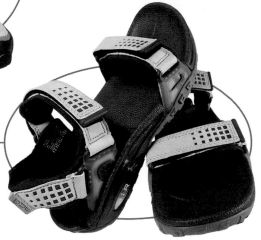

The discomfort of walking in heavy hiking boots in hot weather has inspired a range of trekking sandals that offer support, grip, and flexibility and keep your feet cool in the summer.

keeping warm and dry

It doesn't matter much what you wear for a short walk of 20 minutes or so, as long as you feel comfortable. For longer walks, wear clothes that are loose fitting with elastic waists or non-restrictive materials so that your breathing and your technique are not impaired. Remember: if you don't have to think about your clothes once you are in your stride, then you have it right.

shower and waterproof pants and jacket
Showerproof pants are less cumbersome than waterproof ones, so you can walk in more comfort. They are often made of materials such as Klimate or Gore-Tex or have an inner mesh lining. Lightweight, breathable showerproof and wind-resistant jackets are also ideal. You may need a heavier, waterproof coat if you are walking in exposed places or in wet weather.

reflective strips
If you walk anywhere at night, some of your clothing should have reflective strips or panels.

long-sleeved tops
Current technology has produced excellent materials that maximize warmth, reduce sweating, and ensure comfort when walking. Synthetic materials can trap layers of warm air, absorb the sweat from your skin, and dry quickly if wet. T-shirts made from these materials also tend to be stretchy as well as supportive.

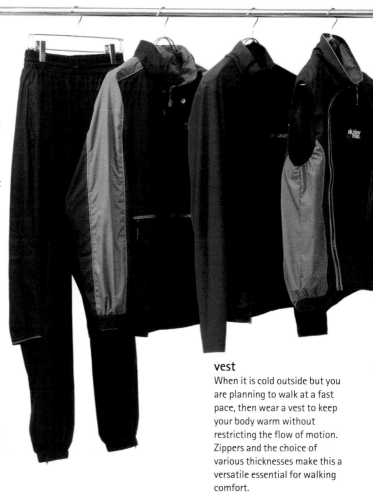

vest
When it is cold outside but you are planning to walk at a fast pace, then wear a vest to keep your body warm without restricting the flow of motion. Zippers and the choice of various thicknesses make this a versatile essential for walking comfort.

winter basics

However cold it feels when you set out, you will get quite warm after a few minutes of brisk walking. Having layers will help control your body temperature, but you don't want to be constantly taking clothes on and off.

Lightweight clothes are best. Clothes such as pants, T-shirts, and fleeces should be loose fitting, apart from the undershirt that is closest to your skin. An undershirt made of synthetic material worn comfortably tight will trap warm air and absorb sweat.

WINTER PROTECTION

Wind and rain should never prevent you from walking. Of course, you can keep warm and dry by staying inside, but improvements in clothing technology keep you just as warm and dry outside. Keeping up with the changing elements during longer walks can be tricky, and it is certainly uncomfortable wearing waterproof clothing when it is not raining. The tricks of the trade, however, are simple:

1 Begin your walk wearing three to four layers of thinner clothes, including a vest for the innermost layer and a waterproof, windproof, and breathable jacket such as Gore-Tex or a waterproof pullover for the top layer. Remember to take a hat, scarf, and gloves for really cold days.

2 Carry a backpack to hold the discarded layers. You need a bag in any case to carry all the other things to make your walk comfortable (see "walking accessories" on pp. 24–25).

3 Take off and put on clothes as needed, if you stop for a rest (when the body temperature drops rapidly) or if the weather changes.

If you have all you need in a smaller fanny pack and prefer not to carry a backpack, you can tie clothes with long sleeves around your waist.

jogging pants

As long as the pants are not too baggy, ordinary tracksuits, whether fleecy or synthetic, are ideal for keeping you warm and comfortable. Cotton pants and jeans are not suitable.

keeping cool

Although it is a great relief when warmer weather arrives, there are other discomforts that come with the summer. The fewer clothes you wear, the more skin-to-skin contact may occur: this can cause painful chafing. Just as important is your exposure to the sun. It is possible to get sunburned even under cloudy skies, and long walks in full sun can cause sunstroke.

SUMMER PROTECTION

Stay cool and safe by taking the following precautions:

1 Always wear sunblock or lotion of at least SPF 15 on your face, neck, ears, and any other exposed parts of your body.

2 Wear a hat with a wide all-around brim.

3 Wear sunglasses with ultraviolet protection to protect your eyes and reduce sun squint.

4 Use Vaseline on parts of your body that may rub and become chafed.

5 If you are likely to encounter insect and plant stings on your walk, then protect yourself with insect repellent, and take antihistamine tablets or cream with you.

6 Keep well hydrated. You are already starting to dehydrate by the time you feel thirsty. Taking frequent sips of water is far better than gulping it down when you are parched (see pp. 24–25 for information on water bottles or pouches).

7 Keep to the shade if possible, and try not to walk during the hottest part of a sunny day, normally between 11 AM and 3 PM.

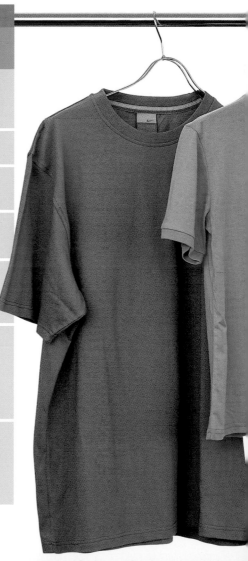

cool clothing

Shorts, light T-shirts, and thinner socks are the main changes you need to make for a summer wardrobe.

shorts

Baggy, longer shorts will keep you cool and protect your legs from too much sun as well as from each other, because they are less likely to rub.

waterproofs

Even in summer, a light waterproof pullover may be necessary for the occasional shower, and you can also use it to sit on when you stop for a rest.

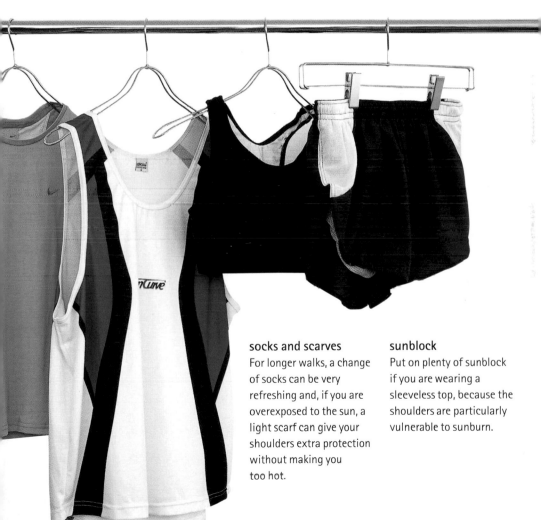

socks and scarves

For longer walks, a change of socks can be very refreshing and, if you are overexposed to the sun, a light scarf can give your shoulders extra protection without making you too hot.

sunblock

Put on plenty of sunblock if you are wearing a sleeveless top, because the shoulders are particularly vulnerable to sunburn.

walking accessories

The last thing you need on a long walk is a large collection of heavy accessories on your back that "may come in handy." Some items, however, will make all the difference in ensuring an enjoyable walk. Some of them are necessities and others, light and small, are worth taking just in case.

If you are race walking, you will travel light, picking up beverages and snacks on the way. However, if you are trekking, hiking, or simply walking on your own, a fanny pack or backpack is ideal to carry all that you need. Leaving your hands free is essential for maintaining your walking technique. Even carrying a fairly light item such as a water bottle or purse can inhibit your arm movements or hunch your shoulders.

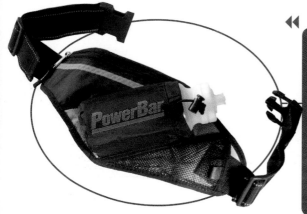

◄◄ water

Plastic water bottles and water pouches with pipes are lightweight; they weigh virtually nothing when empty, and can be carried in your backpack or fanny pack. The type of container you use should depend on the length of your walk and the availability of supplies on the way. Water pouches carry about 4 pints (2 L) compared with the average bottle, which carries 2 pints (1 L). Keep in mind that frequent sipping is encouraged, so don't let the hassle of stopping to get the bottle out of your bag deter you from drinking frequently enough.

compass ►►

A compass is an essential item unless you are on an organized walk. After all, it is often possible to stray off course even when following a route or map. Also take a map of your planned route unless you are keeping to well-signposted roads or are on an organized group walk.

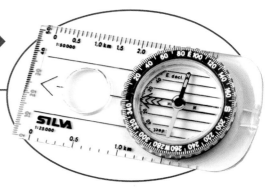

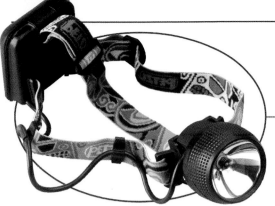

◄◄ flashlight

A flashlight for early nightfall may help you to keep to the route and avoid unseen potholes or tree roots.

sunglasses ►►

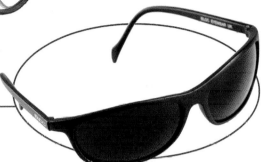

Sunglasses are invaluable in bright sunshine and windy weather, no matter what the season. Make sure you choose a pair that is comfortable, light, and filter out as many harmful UV rays as possible.

necessities (for all weather and seasons)

■ Antihistamine cream or tablets take the pain out of insect and plant stings and can help counter allergic reactions to grass and pollen.

■ Vaseline prevents chafing and blisters.

■ Plasters covering blisters, grazes, and cuts reduce infection and help blisters heal more quickly.

■ A whistle—three blasts is the international emergency signal.

■ Spare socks for wet or warm weather mean that you can change immediately if you have wet or overheated feet. There is nothing worse than wet feet for making you feel cold and miserable.

■ A cell phone or money to make a telephone call is another useful precautionary item.

■ A waterproof pullover for showers, protection when sitting down, or even covering up from the sun.

summer essentials

■ Insect repellent is a necessity in some parts of the world with a large insect population. Mosquito bites are generally harmless, but their bites itch terribly. If you are traveling abroad, find out what insects you might encounter as well as the best methods of preventing and treating their bites.

■ Sunscreen or sunblock is essential and should be reapplied frequently.

cold comfort essentials

■ A hat—more than 70 percent of body heat escapes through the head.

■ Gloves keep your hands warm when the rest of your body is already warmed up.

■ A scarf is essential. For asthmatics, wearing a light, nonwool scarf over your face can warm cold air before it reaches your lungs.

■ A flask of hot drink.

■ A spare T-shirt and socks.

going the distance

If you are planning to take long walks off the beaten track, then make use of the many walking aids available. Price is a good indicator of quality or extra features in this case, so think about what you need before you buy, to avoid paying an extra 10 to 20 percent for something that you will never use.

You can walk at whatever pace you like but you are more likely to meet your goals if you keep track of how your fitness is improving.

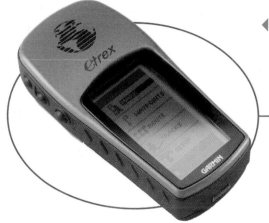

◀◀ satnav or gps

Satellite Navigation Systems (SATNAV) or the Global Positioning System (GPS) are the new orientation systems. They are not cheap, but if you are walking on fairly uncharted territory or simply like the technology, there are ways of using satellite programs to get more out of your walks. Information can also be downloaded onto your computer to chart your progress and record the routes or particular features.

pedometer ▶▶

Are you walking far enough in each session? Pedometers offer a simple and inexpensive guide to the number of steps or the overall distance that you have covered. It is necessary to measure your normal stride over a set distance to calibrate the pedometer, but once set up, it does all the counting for you. You can reset it whenever you like—daily, weekly, or after a defined distance.

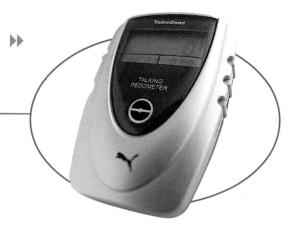

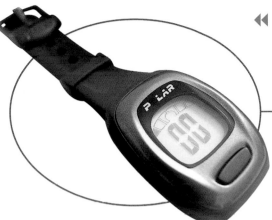

◄◄ heart-rate monitor

Once you have settled into a routine, you can check that you are moving toward your goal by working at the correct training level—your heart rate is the best indication of this. You can wear an electronic monitor to measure your heartbeat, or you can manually assess your heart's activity (see "step to the beat" on pp. 48–49). Heart-rate monitors can vary widely in price. A basic monitor will just measure your heart rate, but many have a watch, a beeping monitor to tell you when you are in the right "training zone," and calorie counters. Some models will hold previous readings so that you can check your progress.

walking poles ►►

When you walk on uneven ground your joints take the strain. Walking sticks, canes, or poles can help minimize the effort. Canes and sticks give a little extra support up the steeper hills and poles help you to maintain your arm movements during the whole walk. Poles are ideal on trails and in fields but are certainly not suitable on roads or stony ground because they need to be planted in a soft surface in order to avoid jarring your body. Walking with poles increases the energy you use by at least a quarter—which is great if you are walking to lose weight! The features to look out for in a walking pole are:

■ Weight and stability—light, sturdy poles are best, made from aluminum, titanium, carbon fiber, or fiberglass.

■ Fixed or telescopic length—if you are taller or shorter than average, a fixed-length pole will strain your back. An adjustable telescopic pole can avoid this, and can be collapsed into a backpack.

■ Antishock features—shock absorbers within the pole, comfortable hand grips, and wrist straps that let you hold the pole quite loosely without losing your grip.

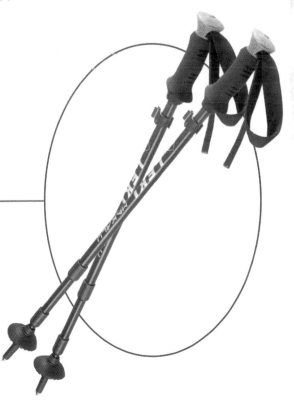

we are what we eat

Nowadays we are constantly made aware of the importance of maintaining a healthy diet and the resulting health problems if we do not. References to fat, refined carbohydrates, calorie requirements, and the way diet contributes to conditions such as diabetes and heart disease can make you feel overwhelmed by the implications of your daily diet.

We all understand the attraction of convenience foods that can simply be put in the microwave or straight into

food and its functions

	FOOD TYPE	WHAT DOES IT DO?
1	CARBOHYDRATE (1 g of carbohydrate is equivalent to 4 kcal)	Provides energy for basic functions and all muscular work (see also "eating well" on pp. 30–31)
2	PROTEIN (1 g of protein is equivalent to 4 kcal)	Supports cell maintenance
3	FAT (1 g of fat is equivalent to 9 kcal)	Provides energy stores for muscular work and the transportation of vitamins
4	WATER	Maintains all bodily functions: our total body weight consists of 50–70 percent water
5	FIBER (soluble and unsoluble)	Helps the stomach and bowels work efficiently
6	TRACE ELEMENTS (vitamins and minerals)	Serve as messengers and catalysts: although tiny amounts are needed, deficiencies cause disease

the mouth—no preparation, no hassle, and no washing up. However, we don't treat our pets and our cars this way. A cat or dog needs a balanced diet and we buy pet food that provides all the necessary nutrients for every meal with no extras. We give the automobile the exact fuel it was designed to use and also ensure it has enough oil changes.

Although we ensure the best health of the things we own, we often think less about what goes into our own bodies. We have become victims of choice.

But it is just as easy to choose a healthy diet—it is not difficult to follow, it doesn't have to cost more money, and it can involve tasty food. So, what does your body need?

WHAT FOODS CONTAIN IT?	HOW MUCH DO YOU NEED?	
Fruits, vegetables, pasta, potatoes, rice, bread, milk	60–70 percent of your dietary intake or about $1/10$ oz a day per lb (6g a day per kg) of body weight	Chocolate, cookies, cakes, and carbonated beverages are all missing from this table. Such foods appeal to your taste buds but are not part of a healthy diet. That doesn't mean you shouldn't eat them; it just means that your body rarely needs them. You can get all you need from other foods, so use these extra sweet, fatty foods for an occasional treat or for a quick energy boost during activity.
Meat, fish, milk, cheese, pulses, nuts, seeds	15 percent of your dietary intake	
Oils, butter, nuts, seeds, avocados, whole milk, cheese	15–25 percent of your dietary intake	
Water is the main ingredient in most drinks but beware of extra calories in sweetened drinks	At least 4 pints (2 L) a day, but more if it is hot or you are very active	
Fruit, vegetables, unrefined carbohydrates such as brown rice and wholemeal bread	A diet rich in unrefined carbohydrates provides sufficient fiber	
Invisible but present in most food; eating a wide range of foods is the best way to get all you need	Requirements vary enormously: vitamins and minerals have recommended daily allowances (RDAs) for the minimum amount required to prevent disease	

eating well

The most available form of carbohydrate as an energy source is a simple sugar. The energy from sugar is released quickly into the bloodstream. A scale called the Glycemic Index (GI) shows how quickly other foods are absorbed compared with sugar. The higher up the scale, the more quickly the food is absorbed. High GI foods can cause a surge of glucose into the blood, which typically provides only temporary satisfaction. Eating a range of lower GI foods keeps blood glucose levels stable—this is good for your heart, reduces the likelihood of excess calories (those not needed for current energy) being converted to fat, and makes you feel fuller for longer.

what is the metabolic rate?

The amount of energy you need to get through the day, before you even think about exercise, is known as the Basal Metabolic Rate (BMR). People who are active not only need more calories for their activity but are also likely to use more calories at rest too.

The built-in problem with most diets is the yo-yo effect. Rapid weight loss may trigger a lowering of the metabolic rate so when normal eating resumes, the weight is regained, and

it is subsequently more difficult to lose. Weight management becomes a lifelong battle, with confidence and enjoyment being the main casualties. Regular exercise can break the vicious circle of yo-yo weight loss.

eating on the move

The blood supply is directed away from the stomach during activity, and digesting food can sometimes cause cramp. However, you will often need to restock your energy while you are walking. Foods that can be digested easily are also easy to eat as you walk—examples are apples, sugary beverages, and low-fat energy bars.

keeping hydrated

■ Prepare beforehand by taking water with you on all walks.

■ Sip fluids frequently rather than waiting until you feel thirsty.

■ Remember that cool fluids are more effective for rehydration, so you will need to drink more hot fluids for the same hydration level.

■ If you are eating dried snacks, such as energy bars or raisins, drink extra fluid.

■ All fluid lost through sweat needs replacing—with a little bit extra. Weigh yourself before and after to

much replacement fluid you need (1 lb [0.5 kg] of weight is equivalent to 1 pint [0.5 L] of fluid).

■ Drink plenty after your walk. Check the color of your urine—it should be pale yellow when you are hydrated.

keeping energy levels up

How and when you eat is just as important as what you eat. Graze, eating small snacks regularly, or eat a meal every three to four hours. Choose carbohydrates rather than foods rich in fat or too much protein, and drink plenty of water beforehand to stave off thirst.

HOW TO LOSE WEIGHT

■ Change one or two eating habits a week rather than going on a drastic diet. Fill in a food diary to keep track.

■ Avoid foods that fill you up but leave you craving for more half an hour later.

■ Aim to reduce your calorie intake by no more than 200 calories a day.

■ Increase your activity levels to burn 500 calories more a day—a 5-mile (8-km) walk.

■ Do not weigh yourself more than once a week, and bear in mind that the muscle you are building weighs more than the fat you are losing—your scales will not recognize this.

preparing for a marathon

By the time you are ready to walk 26 miles (42 km), you will have a good idea of which foods you prefer and how often you need to eat to keep up the pace. There are also some extra things you need to take into account for your first event. Even though you are not "racing," you may feel nervous before you start. Most of those nerves will disappear quickly but they can affect how well you have eaten or drunk beforehand. If your nerves affect your stomach, you may temporarily lose your appetite. Guard against this by making sure that your food intake during the week before the event is well organized: plenty of unrefined carbohydrates, adequate protein, and not too much fat.

1 the week before
Carbohydrate is the best food for energy, so pasta, bread, and rice dishes should be the mainstay, with tomato-based sauces, grilled chicken, lentils, and plenty of fruit and vegetables as accompaniments.

2 the night before
Pasta is excellent in preparation for walking as well as for running events and for good reasons—it is easy to cook, easy to digest, and can be made extra tasty with just a few ingredients. Tomatoes, cheese, and herbs are the classic ingredients.

3 the morning of the marathon
If you don't feel hungry on the morning of the event because of nerves, have some dried bread, rice cakes with juice, or tea to settle your stomach.

4 during the walk
Although you may find plenty of water stations on the route, trying out snacks that you have not had before is not a good idea. Take along your own tried-and-tested snacks, and aim to eat or drink at least 100 calories for each hour that you walk.

5 after the walk
Eating within 2 hours of any long walk is essential to restore your energy levels and minimize muscle soreness. A combination of carbohydrate and protein is ideal, such as a tuna sandwich or a bowl of cereal with low-fat milk. Continue to drink plenty of fluids, but avoid alcohol.

warming up, cooling down 1

Walking over uneven ground can increase the risk of twisting an ankle, especially if your ankles are weak or you have suffered sprains in the past (see "Proprioception," p. 38). Curved roads, hard paving-stone surfaces, or cobbles can also place greater strain on the muscles. Walk on a variety of surfaces, such as grass and asphalt, and try to avoid curved roads that favor one side.

Walking is one of the safest activities you can do and has the least risk of injury. However, failing to warm up and cool down or pushing yourself too hard, too quickly may make you feel unnecessarily stiff and sore.

beat the muscle blues

Always warm up by walking slowly at first, and if you are particularly stiff, especially in the morning, stretch out the calves, hamstrings, and thighs after walking for about 10 minutes. Don't stretch before you start, because cold muscles are more prone to tearing. When you are near the end of your walk, slow down for the last 5 minutes

or so to allow your heart rate to come down gradually and to reduce soreness in your muscles. When you get home, have a drink of water and then stretch out the main muscle groups. Hold (never bounce) each stretch for at least 15 seconds.

Breathe comfortably as you stretch, and don't hold your breath. The muscle being stretched should feel taut but not painful. Get into a good routine by always repeating the stretch on the other leg before starting the next stretch. The eight stretches that follow will reduce any tightness from walking and will act as an early warning to prevent you from storing up problems.

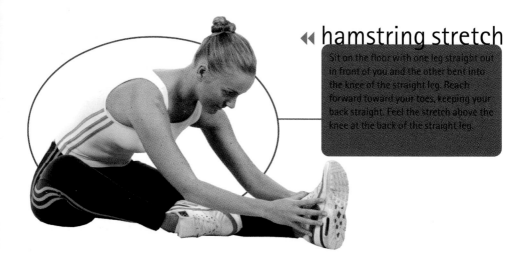

◀◀ hamstring stretch

Sit on the floor with one leg straight out in front of you and the other bent into the knee of the straight leg. Reach forward toward your toes, keeping your back straight. Feel the stretch above the knee at the back of the straight leg.

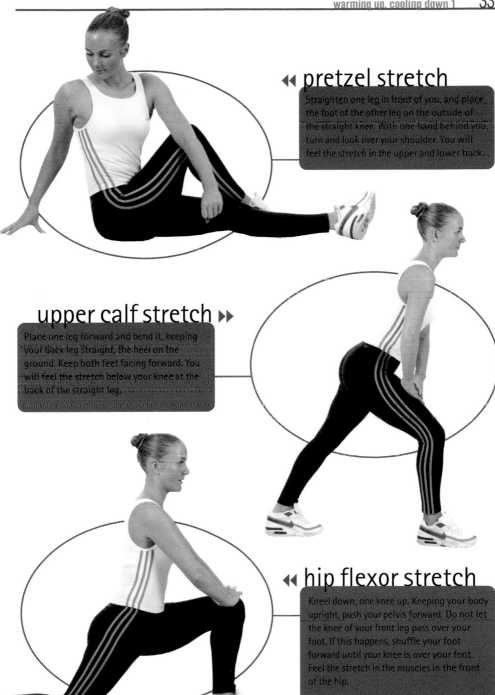

◂◂ pretzel stretch

Straighten one leg in front of you, and place the foot of the other leg on the outside of the straight knee. With one hand behind you, turn and look over your shoulder. You will feel the stretch in the upper and lower back.

upper calf stretch ▸▸

Place one leg forward and bend it, keeping your back leg straight, the heel on the ground. Keep both feet facing forward. You will feel the stretch below your knee at the back of the straight leg.

◂◂ hip flexor stretch

Kneel down, one knee up. Keeping your body upright, push your pelvis forward. Do not let the knee of your front leg pass over your foot. If this happens, shuffle your foot forward until your knee is over your foot. Feel the stretch in the muscles in the front of the hip.

warming up, cooling down 2

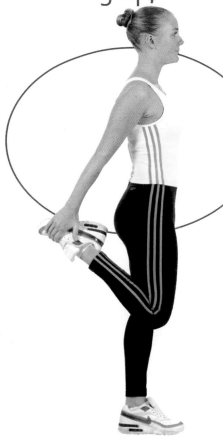

◀◀ quadriceps stretch

Pull one foot behind you, toward, but not touching, your buttock. Keep both hips facing forward and your knees together. Feel the stretch down the front of the thigh. To increase the stretch, push your pelvis forward slightly.

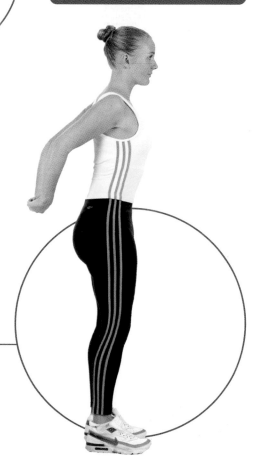

pectoral stretch ▶▶

Clasp your hands lightly behind your back, which gently pushes the shoulder blades together. Breathe easily and gently push your chest out. Feel the stretch across the top of the chest.

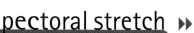

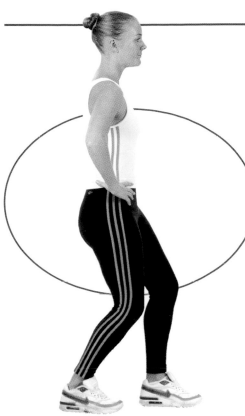

◀◀ lower calf stretch

With one leg bent, bring your other leg forward. Keep both feet flat and facing forward. You should feel the stretch in the lower calf of the back leg just above the heel.

shin stretch ▶▶

Stand on one leg, supporting yourself on a wall if necessary. Stretch one leg out in front of you and point the toes downward and inward to feel the stretch on the outside of the shin. Then point them outward for the same length of time to stretch the inner shin.

resting

If you are training hard, you need more than just a few stretches if you expect your body to keep up the pace. Regular rest and relaxation (R & R) days are essential to allow the body to recover and get stronger. Rest at least once a week by doing a very gentle walk or possibly nothing at all. Even if you don't feel stiff, a lighter session should follow a hard hill or speed session to prevent overtraining and reduce muscle damage. You may be eager to advance your training, but you won't achieve this if you don't rest. Regular easy days, weeks, and months will make you fitter and stronger much more quickly.

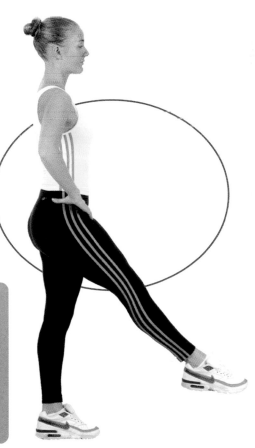

walking form

To get the most out of power walking, your technique is paramount. Using the correct technique may feel odd at first, especially if you are only used to walking when you are shopping or taking short trips, in which case you will not have noticed any problems due to poor posture when walking. When you feel ready to improve your walking technique, work on one area of the body at a time.

home training

Certain exercises can be done at home to improve strength and to help you overcome any injuries. This series of exercises will strengthen a range of muscles and can be progressed as you get fitter.

Do these exercises when you are warm after having walked. Do not do them while cold. Also, do not use them if you have been told that you have high blood pressure.

WORKING ON WALKING

FEET FIRST

The foot is a complex limb that has 26 bones, 33 connecting joints, 107 ligaments, and 19 muscles; its strength lies in the combination of rigidity (from the bones) and flexibility (from the muscles and ligaments). When the foot lands on the ground, the heel should strike first. The foot rolls slightly inward as the heel lifts and all the weight ends up on the ball of the foot. Just before it leaves the ground for the next step, the big toe pushes down. If there are variations in this gait—for example, not landing first on the heel or failing to roll smoothly through to the ball of the foot—then other muscles have to compensate and can get strained.

BACK AND TORSO

Stand tall with your stomach pulled up, your pelvis slightly tilted forward and your shoulders held lightly back in a neutral posture.

Years of incorrect walking may now feel quite normal. When you start walking taller and straighter, weak and underused muscles will fire up and may cause discomfort. Persevere—it is worth it. Tight muscles in any part of the body can cause postural changes that may only show up when damage has already been done.

Walking puts considerable emphasis on the muscles attached to the pelvis. Tight hip flexors or hamstrings can also place great strain on the lower back. To avoid strain, build up your walking gradually, keep your stride to a comfortable length, and make sure that you stretch after each session. If you normally walk carrying a briefcase or purse on one side, you may have developed a lopsided walk. If you notice tightness down one side only, you may need professional help to correct it.

WORKING THE CORE: ELBOWS AND KNEES

Lie down on the floor on your front (on a mat or carpet). Rest your elbows and forearms on the floor, with your elbows under the shoulders. Straighten out your body and legs, rest your knees on the floor, hold in your stomach, relax your hands, and keep your body straight. Take care not to arch your lower back. Keep your chin at a right angle to your chest so that you are looking at your wrists or hands. Hold the position for 5–30 seconds. Don't forget to breathe regularly while maintaining the position.

You can advance this exercise as you feel ready by using the same basic position with various subsidiary positions.

- Hands and feet
- Hands and one foot, with the other one resting on top, alternating the position
- Hands and one foot held out to the side

- Elbows and feet
- Elbows and one foot, alternating the position
- Elbows and one foot held out to the side

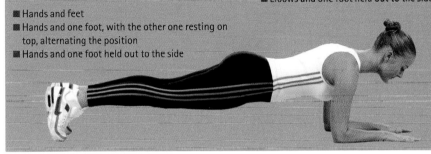

ARMS AND SHOULDERS

Your upper limbs and shoulders should feel comfortable, and walking with your hands free will allow maximum relaxation. Bend the arms at a 90-degree angle, curl the hands lightly as though you are holding precious egg shells, and move them in a fairly small arc from the side of the waist to the chest, each arm in opposition with the leg. The arms and legs are always in step: the faster you pump your arms, the faster your legs can go. Don't use weights to increase your upper body strength while you are walking, because they can strain the shoulders and joints and affect your gait. If you want to get stronger, use light dumbbells at home, or even use household items such as dried foods and bottles as cheap alternatives.

HEAD AND NECK

When you are walking, you want to see not only where you are going but also what you are about to tread on. Keeping your head upright, with your eyes focused a little distance ahead, allows you to do both. Walking with your head down, especially if you are carrying a backpack, will strain the neck and shoulders. When you have finished your walk, gently move your head in a semicircle from shoulder to shoulder a few times to ease any tension.

STRIDE LENGTH

A comfortable stride length will help you enjoy your walks without overstraining. As you get fitter, your stride may get longer, although long strides do not necessarily mean a faster pace. The rate at which your legs move is a better indicator of speed, and this will definitely increase as you get fitter.

walking wounded

Injuries in most parts of the body, from muscle strains to tendon and ligament sprains, are accompanied by swelling as blood rushes to the affected area. Because this can cause more damage to the tissues, the main point of first aid is to reduce this swelling and prevent further damage that may hamper recovery.

When you start walking to get fit, you may find it difficult to know the difference between soreness caused by unaccustomed activity and real injury. Follow the first-aid principles given here at the first sign of pain, and see a doctor if the pain does not fade after a couple of days.

exercises to overcome injury

proprioception

Perform this exercise for an injured ankle:

1 Balance on the uninjured foot alone first, holding on to something for support.
2 Try to balance without support.
3 Repeat the exercise, this time with your eyes closed.
4 Bearing in mind what your good foot can do, repeat steps 1 through 3 on the injured foot.

knee tracking

If you feel pain in your kneecap or the outside of your knee, do the following exercise:

Sit down on a chair or the floor with your legs stretched out in front of you. Use your hands for support. Squeeze the thigh muscle and make the knee flatten. The heel may lift off the floor, but this is not important. Turn your foot outward, and supporting your back with your hands behind you, lift your leg 2–3 in (5–7.5 cm) off the floor. Repeat this small up-and-down movement between 10 and 20 times.

ICER treatment

Ice the affected area with an ice pack or a packet of frozen peas wrapped in a cloth. Leave the ice on for no longer than 10 minutes, and repeat at least three times a day.

Compress the affected area with a bandage, particularly for the first 24 hours. Check that fingers or toes do not turn blue because of an over-tight dressing. If you have diabetes or any loss of sensation, avoid using compression.

Elevate the arm or leg to reduce the blood supply to the area. Check that the circulation is not impaired.

Rest the affected limb. If the injury is not serious, a couple of days off will probably be adequate treatment. If the injury takes longer to heal, you can use other activities to maintain your fitness (see "Cross training" on pp. 44–45).

remedies for five common walking injuries

INJURY	POSSIBLE CAUSE	TREATMENT AND PREVENTION
ACHILLES TENDON INJURY	Caused by hard surfaces, overtraining, heel tabs rubbing, or the Achilles tendon shortening through the wearing of high heels.	■ Follow ICER. ■ Vary your walking surface and heel size, build up the intensity gradually, and check that your shoes have a soft heel tab. ■ Practice the lower calf stretch.
ANKLE INJURY	Recovery from injured ankles can leave tight scar tissue, vulnerability to further tears and weakness, and loss of balance awareness.	■ Retrain the balancing senses (see "Proprioception" on p. 38).
KNEE PAIN	Often due to gait but can be caused by tight or unbalanced muscles in other areas, such as the back, buttocks, and quadriceps in the thigh.	■ Follow ICER. ■ Strengthen your quadriceps (use "knee tracking" opposite). ■ If caused by muscle imbalance or tight iliotibial (IT) band, see treatment and stretches on pp. 32–35. Check with a physiotherapist if self-treatment fails.
SHIN SPLINTS	Overpronation or shortened tendons in the toes cause the shin muscles to overcontract. Most common in beginners or when changing terrain.	■ Follow ICER. ■ Consider orthotics (shoe inserts) for overpronation. ■ Pay attention to shin and calf stretches. ■ Strengthen the shin muscle by running or walking up steps, and stretch the calf muscle with a standard calf stretch.
TIGHTNESS in any part of the legs	Overstriding, overtraining, lack of warm up and cool down, or just walking too much, too quickly.	■ Follow ICER. ■ See pp. 32–35 on how to warm up and cool down. ■ See the section on walking form on pp. 36–37 and follow the training schedules to prevent overdoing it.

Sports massage, physiotherapist treatment, or specialist podiatrists can identify problems in the early stages, prevent muscle damage, and promptly treat injuries. Look at it like an automobile service: don't wait for a breakdown before you go to the garage.

motivation

Even avid walkers can feel like putting today's walk off until tomorrow. A day off will not do you any harm, but if your motivation is lagging, these pages will help you to stay on track.

realistic goals

You are more likely to give up trying to reach a goal if the goal is unreasonable. Revisit your goal, and make sure it is still SMART (see pp. 12–13). If you are feeling temporarily demotivated, use the checklist on the next page to find out why.

what works best for you?

If you feel too tired to go for a walk after work, you may need to plan your walks for another part of the day, such as lunchtime or the early morning, both good for keeping you alert all day. However, your walks should suit your daily routine—if you are full of energy in the morning, then stick to morning walks, or if you are more active in the evening, walking then may suit your natural rhythm better. Longer walks can then be scheduled on the weekends to suit you and your family and friends.

positive thinking

Once you have made it outside the door, it is generally easy to keep walking for as long as you planned. If you are not in the mood, however, negative thoughts can creep in and undermine your motivation. The two most common negative thoughts are:

ten tips to stay on course

1
Go somewhere new—a new route will challenge you, and new sights are always interesting.

2
Join a walking group—if there isn't a local group, think about setting one up yourself.

3
Make your own map—see how much you have taken in of a region that you know. Does it match the reality? Have fun comparing yours with an actual map.

4
Take a friend's dog with you—all dogs relish the idea of a walk.

5
Take a day or two off—although you need to exercise regularly, you don't have to exercise every single day.

■ **I don't have time for this today.**
Time away from your normal routine can recharge your batteries and help you to work out solutions to problems.

■ **My legs are too short/long/fat to walk fast.**
There is no perfect walker's body, so just enjoy this most natural of movements to the fullest.

avoiding the pitfalls

■ **Are you progressing slower than you want to?**

■ **Are you afraid that you aren't going to meet your goal?**
When you are working on building up your fitness and strength, improvements are not always measured in a straight upward curve. There is a tendency to make rapid progress at first, followed by a plateau, followed by a move up to the next level, followed by another plateau and so on. This process allows the body time to adapt and consolidate the improvements. So be patient, enjoy following the program, and you will reach your goal.

■ **Are you aching more than usual?**
■ **Are you too tired?**
Aching or tiredness could be caused by the process of adapting to the new regime. When you push yourself too hard, too quickly, your body doesn't have time to recover, and the result is fatigue and soreness. If you are training hard, you still need to have lighter walking sessions and days of rest. Also, check that you are eating and drinking enough: one symptom of dehydration is fatigue, and if you have cut back your calories at the same time, you may not be eating enough protein and carbohydrates to feed your muscles.

■ **Are you bored with the same old routes?**
We all need routine in our lives but variety also keeps us alert and challenged. If you do the same walk each day, try a different route. Also, if your walk coincides with a social event or favorite TV program, rethink your schedule. The walk is important, but so is taking the occasional day off to do something else.

6 Marshall at an event—volunteers are always needed, and you will be reminded of why you took up walking.

7 Inspire others—telling friends or acquaintances what walking does for you will strengthen your own resolve, while hopefully inspiring them.

8 Buy a walking kit—walking clothes, equipment, or new route maps can give you the inspiration to walk as well as a bit of retail therapy.

9 Think positively—when you have a negative thought, look for the positive option to replace it.

10 Challenge yourself—set yourself a silly goal, such as walking up every set of stairs or escalators on the way home from work.

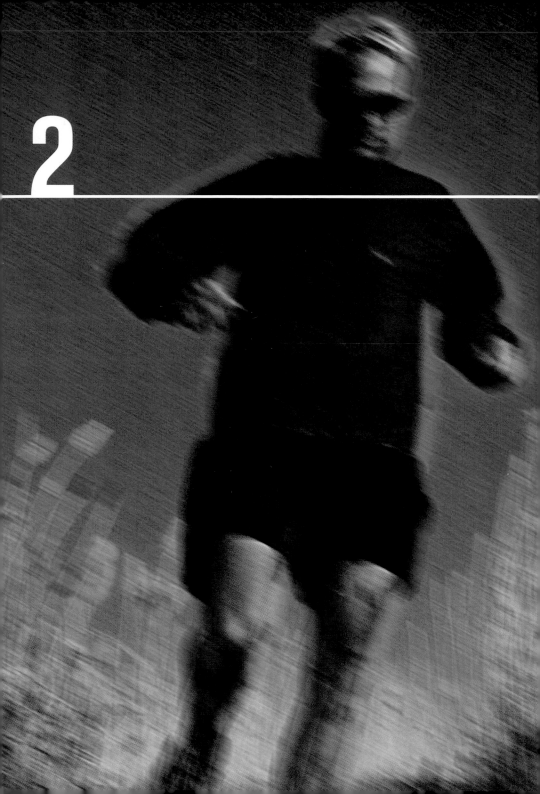

2

training schedules

This chapter looks at training schedules from complete
beginner (level 1) to marathon walker (level 6). The path to
success is marked out with signposts. As far as power
walking is concerned, that means signposts for checking
that you are moving in the right direction at the right pace.
But just as signposts tell you what is up ahead, they don't
say that you have to go there—so you can deviate from the
route, pause to look at the scenery, or go at a pace that
suits you. Following a schedule will at least ensure that you
arrive at your destination at some point. The schedules
here will guide you to your chosen goal. They also point out
the interesting scenery you may pass, explain why
deviations are sometimes a good idea, and provide a map
when you have lost your way. So enjoy your journey.

following the schedules

four golden nuggets

1

To reduce the risk of injury, start and end your walk at a slower pace than the main part. Five minutes at each end is normally enough, unless it is particularly cold, in which case it should be longer. Always stretch out once you have finished (see pp. 32–35).

2

Follow the schedule. The schedule will progressively increase in pace, intensity, and length. If you have a break of more than a week, restart where you left off rather than jumping to the following week.

3

Listen to your body. If you feel aches and pains, it is likely for a very good reason. Either you have overdone it or you have strained something. Rest will help, but see a doctor or specialist for any problem that doesn't resolve itself within a few days.

4

Cross train. You need a range of sessions to build strength and stamina. Brisk, steady, up-and-down inclines and days of complete rest are both essential. If you want even more variety, you could try other activities, such as cycling or swimming.

Any increase in activity will improve your fitness, but following a schedule will yield the fastest results. Combine the training schedules that follow with the golden nuggets on the left, and you have all you need to apply the principles to your own training plan. Wherever you are in the schedule, basic rules ensure that you protect yourself from injury and don't stray too far from the path. You will find all the basic warm-up and walking techniques in the previous chapter. Reread these as you move through the program to help you get the most benefit from your training.

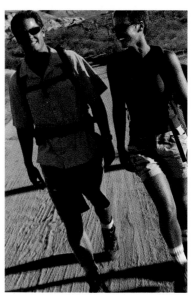

training sessions

Training sessions vary enormously, and this is not just to keep participants interested, but also because different sessions promote every aspect of strength, endurance, and speed that you need to develop. These elements cannot be developed by repeating the same walk. The outlines given here will help you understand what aspect you are working on and what you are hoping to achieve.

brisk walks ▶▶

Brisk walks are the training staple. Sessions from 30–60 minutes will improve strength and stamina. The pace you maintain on these walks will give you a good idea of how fast you will cover the longer distances as your fitness improves.

speed work ▶▶

The speed work session pushes you to the limits of your speed ability. Maintain your walking form as you build up sprints from 30 seconds to 5 minutes with a recovery period of 3 to 5 minutes. Repeat 4 to 10 times until you can maintain the faster pace with hardly any time at the recovery pace.

long, steady walks ▶▶

Any walk of more than an hour should be seen as an opportunity to maintain a fairly constant pace, even over hills or uneven terrain. It is imperative to spend time on your feet: shorter sessions are no substitute for this part of the program.

hill sessions ▶▶

Climbing down a hill is just as hard work as climbing up one: it just works different muscles and feels a bit easier on your heart and lungs. Vary the inclines and aim to walk at the same pace up hills as you do on the flat. In this way, you will build up your strength and stamina.

opportunity ▶▶

Every time you get the chance for a quick walk during the day, practice your technique, walking tall or shortening your stride to achieve the maximum number of steps.

how the training levels work

This section outlines a range of schedules designed to train you to achieve your goal. You can start at whatever level your current fitness allows. Each schedule is harder than the previous one, with the first level aimed at those people who have not been regularly active for the last year.

your call

The schedules are here to guide rather than dominate. They will lead you

1 complete beginner	**2** starter level	**3** refresher level
## pages 52–55	## pages 56–59	## pages 60–65
Complete beginner level is for walkers who can walk only 5 minutes comfortably. This first schedule includes 5 days a week of gentle or brisker walks of 20–30 minutes.	Starter level is for leisure walkers who are already walking at a moderate pace for at least 30 minutes during the day. Use this schedule to:	Refresher level is for those who have had a break in their program or who can walk for 45 minutes at $3^1/_2$ mph (5.6 km/h) for at least 4 days a week. Use this schedule to train to achieve:
■ This level will get you walking for 30 minutes continuously at a brisk pace.	■ walk continuously for 3 miles (4.8 km) at a good pace	■ improvements in fitness (4-week training cycles)
■ Drop in or out of this schedule if you have a break for longer than a month.	■ increase your pace and distances.	■ a walk of 4 hours with short stops.

toward a goal, but they are also aimed at a wide range of people. Because of this, it is important to relate them to your own situation. Plan to modify the schedule as necessary so that you can keep walking and stay free from injury: always see a doctor if you are concerned about any pain or injury.

take your time

Work through the levels at your own pace and drop down to the previous level if it feels too hard. Although these schedules are challenging, they are not competitions or exercises to see how far you can push yourself before you reach exhaustion. So listen to your body and your mind – if you are tired, rest.

4 intermediate level	**5** upper level	**6** advanced level
pages 66–71	**pages 72–79**	**pages 80–87**
regular walkers who can walk 3 miles (4.8 km) in less than an hour 5 days a week. This program will start off those who wish to train for a marathon. Also use to train for:	experienced walkers or trekkers who are able to walk every day for 1 hour at a minimum of 3^1/$_2$ mph (5.6 km/h) (see pp. 72–79). Use this schedule to train for:	walkers who spend at least 1 day a week walking for 2 hours and 1 hour every other day at 3^1/$_2$ mph (5.6 km/h). Use this schedule to train for:
■ improvements in fitness (4-week training cycles)	■ improvements in fitness (4-week training cycles)	■ improvements in fitness (4-week training cycles)
■ a walk of 11 or more miles (17.7 km or more) in 3 hours on flat terrain	■ a 6-mile (9.6-km) event walk	■ a weeklong trekking expedition
■ a half-day trek (4–5 hours) over rough terrain	■ a daylong trek (8–9 hours) over rough terrain.	■ a charity event marathon
■ a 6-mile (9.6-km) event walk.		■ a marathon event walk.

step to the beat

A heart-rate monitor will give you moment-by-moment readings on how hard you are working. However, if you prefer just to wear one occasionally (or not at all), you can also match up how you are feeling with a specific reading, and use that as guidance to check that you are working at the right level.

To know your target heart rate, you will need to know your maximum. If you are more than 20 percent overweight or a beginner, it is best to use the approximate formula below to estimate your maximum:

214 – (0.8 x age) for men

209 – (0.9 x age) for women

For example, a 30-year-old man might have a rate of:

0.8 x 30 = 24

214 – 24 =190

INTENSITY	HR % OF WHR	RPE (1–10)	TYPE OF ACTIVITY
Very low intensity	35–45	2–4	Standing
Low intensity	45–55	4–5	Strolling, doing housework
Moderate activity	55–75	6–7	Brisk walking
High intensity	75-85	8–9	Walking uphill

Key: HR = heart rate; WHR = working heart rate; RPE = rate of perceived exertion
(Note: RPE is a completely subjective method of evaluating how you feel.)

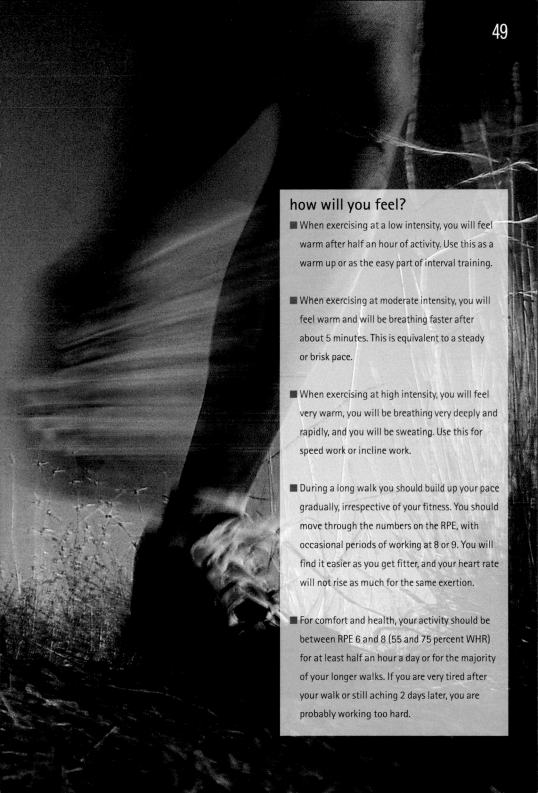

how will you feel?

■ When exercising at a low intensity, you will feel warm after half an hour of activity. Use this as a warm up or as the easy part of interval training.

■ When exercising at moderate intensity, you will feel warm and will be breathing faster after about 5 minutes. This is equivalent to a steady or brisk pace.

■ When exercising at high intensity, you will feel very warm, you will be breathing very deeply and rapidly, and you will be sweating. Use this for speed work or incline work.

■ During a long walk you should build up your pace gradually, irrespective of your fitness. You should move through the numbers on the RPE, with occasional periods of working at 8 or 9. You will find it easier as you get fitter, and your heart rate will not rise as much for the same exertion.

■ For comfort and health, your activity should be between RPE 6 and 8 (55 and 75 percent WHR) for at least half an hour a day or for the majority of your longer walks. If you are very tired after your walk or still aching 2 days later, you are probably working too hard.

stronger, faster, quicker

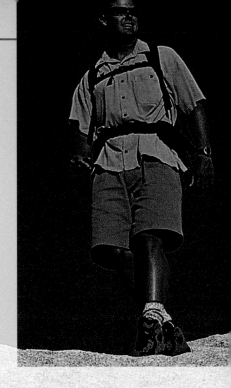

You might think that there couldn't be a special technique for walking faster. However, there are specific sessions designed to increase your speed and these are known as interval or repetition sessions. By allowing yourself a recovery period in between each "interval," you will be able to maintain a faster pace than normal and build up your stamina and speed. And it takes as little as one session a week to change a leisurely pace into a continuous speedy pace.

But, before you even think about increasing your speed, you need to be able to walk at a brisk pace for 30 minutes without feeling out of breath. The first interval session will feel hard, but don't panic—that's to be expected. You will soon get used to it, and it will make your normal pace feel like a breeze.

types of interval

The definition of interval exercise is simple: periods of higher intensity followed by rest or recovery. It doesn't all have to be pure speed: you can do hill intervals or timed intervals, or you can simply work at a higher intensity for part of your normal, longer walks. If your walk is over hilly terrain, the climb up a hill may be intense but the climb down, though you are still working your leg muscles, is a chance to recover and get your breath back. Short bursts of speed or climbing will improve speed alone, whereas longer bouts will work

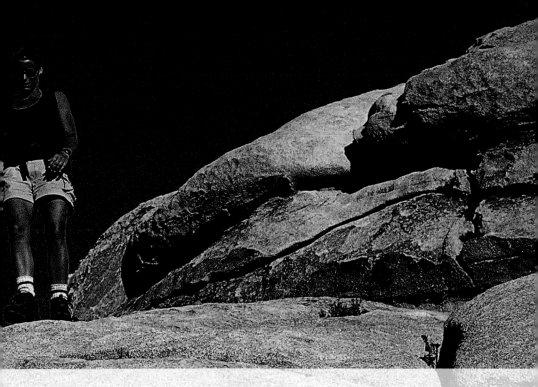

on your endurance as well. Aim for short bursts and long recovery times for speed, and longer intense periods of 5 to 10 minutes with shorter recovery periods of 1 to 2 minutes for endurance and speed. You can have your interval and rest period start/stop locations defined by intersecting streets, every fourth streetlight, or any other geographical feature.

event walking

The rules of event walking are straightforward: one foot must be in contact with the ground at all times. This rule does stop people from running, but extra speed can still be achieved by swinging the hips from side to side. Although this may look a little strange to the uninitiated, the speed that experienced walkers gain in this way is quite remarkable, with the pace often equaling that of a runner.

how hard should it feel?

Once you reach a comfortable level of fitness and can walk continuously without feeling breathless, an interval session will push you to make a greater effort, reflected by your breathing and level of warmth. You should be able to recover within the given time and feel that you are putting in the same extra effort for all intervals. This method of training can improve your fitness faster than just walking briskly, and it will teach you to maintain your technique when you pick up the pace.

1

complete beginner

Level 1 will suit all those who are completely new to power walking. By the time you have worked through this schedule, you will be able to walk for 30 minutes continuously without getting out of breath. You will have begun to experience the joy and benefits of regular walking and will know that you can do it.

If you start at the beginning of the schedule and realize that it is too easy, you can skip the first couple of weeks or just work through the first schedule more quickly. But don't be too enthusiastic and jump in too far ahead, because no matter how easy you find it, your body still needs to adapt to regular activity. Parts of the body take

different times to strengthen and adjust to new demands. Beginners are the most prone to injuries because their enthusiasm often overtakes their body's abilities. Joints are particularly susceptible to injury during the early phase of a new training regimen: you often don't realize you have overdone it until the next day or even the day after that. Strong, safe buildings are built on good foundations, and this schedule provides the best materials for building the foundations for a lifetime of regular and enjoyable walking.

adding new challenges

When you can walk for 30 minutes continuously over a distance of

too easy?

If you've always been active, although maybe not in a formal way, your body may cope well with the program, in which case you may want to move through the schedules more swiftly. You still need time to adapt, however, so aim to increase the length of time you spend walking rather than speeding up too much in these initial weeks. (See p. 55 for safe ways to increase the pace if you are fitter than you thought.)

level 1 schedule

To keep it safe and simple, do the same session throughout each week. Three to four sessions a week are ideal, allowing for a break of about a day in between. Use this time to put into practise what you learned from the first chapter. Concentrate on your breathing: it should be deep and even, expanding your abdomen as well as your chest. Pay attention to your walking technique, and consider anything that may need attention. For example, are you hunched, clenched, or leaning too far forward?

This is the time to work out how to use any technical equipment you have bought. If you build up the exercise level gradually, your muscles may feel tight but they shouldn't feel sore. Get into the routine of stretching from the outset to build good habits. Underused muscles will creak and complain a bit, but these pains should disappear after the first week or two. If they don't, consult a doctor to ensure that nothing is seriously wrong.

2 miles (3.2 km), use the next few weeks to increase the number of times you walk. When you can walk briskly for 30 minutes three times a week, you are ready to start level 2.

When you can walk for 15 minutes twice a day, aim to add one minute until you are doing an extra five minutes for each walk. Start at week 5 or, if this is too much, drop back a week.

WEEK 1
Walk briskly for 1 minute and slowly for 1 minute. Repeat 10 times.

WEEK 2
Walk briskly for 3 minutes and slowly for 1 minute. Repeat 7 times.

WEEK 3
Walk briskly for 5 minutes and slowly for 1 minute. Repeat 5 times.

WEEK 4
Walk briskly for 8 minutes and slowly for 2 minutes. Repeat 3 times.

WEEK 5
Walk briskly for 6 minutes and slowly for 1 minute. Then walk briskly for 10 minutes and gently for 2 minutes.

WEEK 6
Walk briskly for 10 minutes and slowly for 1 minute. Repeat 3 times.

▸▸ week 3—how's it going?

Can you walk and talk? Are the gentle walks long enough for recovery? Are you walking comfortably? If so, you are fine to move on to week 4. If the answer to any of the questions is "no," then see p. 54. If you feel you could go much faster or for a longer time and you are not tired, move on to week 7.

week 6—how's it going?

Does 10 minutes of continuous walking make you breathless? If so, go back to week 4 or 5, whichever feels comfortable. If you are ready to go further, go on to week 8, but don't skip any more weeks—remember the adaptation process avoiding injury makes it worth the wait.

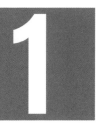

complete beginner

it's too hard!

The dropout rate for people new to exercise can be as high as 50 percent. The main reason for this, apart from unrealistic expectations (see pp. 40–41), is that it feels too hard. And, of course, it will be hard if your body is not ready. Experienced walkers don't push themselves too hard, too soon, and as a result they aren't permanently laid up with injuries. That is because they have worked slowly and steadily to get to a point where they can enjoy walking throughout the year on all terrain.

You may have told yourself that walking would be easy and may be worried that if this feels too hard you must be really unfit. If you are convinced that walking is the best exercise in the world, then why does it feel so difficult? Power walking for fitness is more than just walking out to the car, the store, or across the road. It requires strength, stamina, and speed, and these you have to acquire gradually. Your body certainly has the capability, but that doesn't mean it is ready for it all at once. So if it is harder than you imagined, remind yourself why you started, think about how long you have allocated to reach your goal, and don't forget that the best things in life do take time.

WEEK 7

Walk briskly for 12 minutes and slowly for 2 minutes.
Then walk briskly for 15 minutes and gently for 2 minutes.

WEEK 8

Walk briskly for 14 minutes and slowly for 1 minute.
Then walk briskly for 17 minutes and gently for 2 minutes.

WEEK 9

Walk briskly for 16 minutes and slowly for 1 minute.
Then walk briskly for 20 minutes and gently for 2 minutes.

week 9—how's it going?

Are you finding that this is a breeze and you are impatient to walk for the whole time with no breaks? If you have no aches, pains or breathlessness, then go ahead. If you are not so sure, have an extra rest after day 2 of week 10 and see how you feel. You can always break up the 30-minute brisk walk with a gentle pace every 10 minutes or so.

Don't be too proud to stay on the first or second week program until it feels comfortable. If you are looking to lose weight, keeping active with walking will help you do that, and it will also help you to become fitter and faster.

Move on to the next week when you feel ready: that is, when your breathing is comfortable and you are not aching the next day. Look back at the tips to stay motivated (see pp. 40–41) and don't give up.

moving on faster

If it feels comfortable and you have no joint pain, it is a sign that you are ready to do this schedule in seven or eight weeks instead of ten. Miss out every third or fourth week but always be willing to drop back if it feels too fast—don't push yourself beyond your capabilities. Alternatively, you can increase the number of sessions you do each week, but make sure you have at least one day of rest in each week.

aches...?

Carrying a bag on one shoulder, a heavy backpack, hunching the shoulders, or having round shoulders and a tilted-back head all lead to neck and shoulder ache. To counter this problem, only carry the bare essentials evenly distributed across both shoulders. Also, look at your walking technique (see pp. 36–37) and work on keeping your upper body relaxed.

WEEK
10 DAILY SCHEDULE

DAY 1: Walk briskly for 10 minutes and slowly for 1 minute. Then walk briskly for 22 minutes and slowly for 2 minutes.

DAY 2: Walk briskly for 10 minutes, slowly for 10 minutes, and gently for 5 minutes.

DAY 3: Walk briskly for 10 minutes, slowly for 2 minutes, and briskly for 25 minutes.

DAY 4: Rest.

DAY 5: Walk briskly for 15 minutes and slowly for 1 minute.

DAY 6: Walk briskly for 10 minutes and slowly for 5 minutes. Then briskly for 10 minutes and gently for 5 minutes.

DAY 7: Walk briskly for 30 minutes.

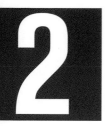

starter level 4 weeks, repeatable

Level 2, which should be repeated over four weeks, is for leisure walkers who are already walking at a moderate pace for at least 30 minutes during the day. This schedule consists of a fitness program and a continuous walk for 3 miles (4.8 km). If you are spreading your 30 minutes of walking throughout the day, this will give you the chance to build up to longer sessions and learn how to pace yourself so that you can keep going.

level 2 fitness schedule

Whether you want to walk in a short- or long-distance event, or go for a trek in the countryside, you should have a basic level of fitness. All you are aiming for at the moment is to walk regularly and make it a regular habit, and any improvements in strength and stamina are a bonus.

WEEK	MONDAY	TUESDAY
1	rest	10 min slow at RPE 5; 3 x 1 min at RPE 8 with 2 min recoveries at RPE 4–5; 10 min at RPE 6–7
CYCLE 2		add 1 repeat
2	rest	10 min slow at RPE 5; 15 min varied pace; 10 min at RPE 6–7
CYCLE 2		add 5 min
3	rest	10 min slow at RPE 5; 4 x 1 1/2 min at RPE 8 with 2 1/2 min recoveries at RPE 4–5; 10 min at RPE 6–7
CYCLE 2		add 30 sec to repeat
4	rest	10 min steady at RPE 6; 2 x 4 min at RPE 8 with 4 min recoveries at RPE 4–5; 4 min at RPE 7
CYCLE 2		add 1 min to repeat

week 4—how's it going?

Take stock: you have been walking for about 3 months now, so you are developing good habits. If you are walking through persistent pains or ignoring an injury that you hope will just go away, it is time to see a doctor. If you are comfortable at the end of week 4 and you want to go on to level 3, start week 5 with the second cycle. If not, or you just want a couple more weeks to settle into it, repeat the first cycle until you feel ready to move on.

rate of exertion

Each session is indicated by:

- an approximate pace—slow, brisk, or fast
- the type of training—steady, inclines, long, or interval techniques
- how hard you should be working—indicated by the RPE rate (see pp. 48–49)

WEDNESDAY	THURSDAY	FRIDAY	SATURDAY	SUNDAY
30 min at RPE 6–7	10 min slow at RPE 5–6; 5 min brisk at RPE 7–8; 10 min slow at RPE 5–6	rest	30 min at RPE 6–7	35 min steady at RPE 6–7
	add 5 min			add 10 min
35 min at RPE 6	10 min slow at RPE 6; 5 min brisk at RPE 7–8; 10 min slow at RPE 6	rest	35 min at RPE 6	45 min steady at RPE 6–7
	add 3 min			add 10 min
40 min at RPE 6	10 min at RPE 6–7; 5 min at RPE 7–8; 10 min at RPE 6–7	rest	35 min at RPE 6	50 min steady at RPE 6–7
	add 4 min			add 15 min
45 min at RPE 6	10 min at RPE 6; 10 min at RPE 7–8; 10 min at RPE 6	rest	35 min at RPE 6	1 hr steady at RPE 6–7
	add 5 min			add 15 min

▲ how's it going?

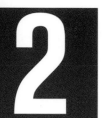

starter 3 miles (4.8 km)

Y ou need to be able to walk at a brisk pace for 30 continuous minutes on at least three days of the week.

week 3—how's it going?

You can get an idea of your 3-mile (4.8-km) time from your time trial.

MPH	MIN PER MILE	3 MILES (4.8 KM)
3¼	18	55 min
3½	17	52 min
3¾	16	48 min
4	15	45 min
4¼	14	43 min
4½	13	40 min
5	12	37 min

If you have planned your first 3-mile (4.8-km) race, then there are only 2 more weeks to go. If you don't feel ready yet, spend another week or two building up to this level.

WEEK	MONDAY	TUESDAY
1	rest	10 min steady at RPE 6–7; 4 x 1 min at RPE 9 with 2 min recoveries at RPE 4–5; 10 min at RPE 6–7
2	rest	10 min at RPE 6–7; 3 x 4 min at RPE 8 with 3 min recoveries at RPE 4–5; 4 min at RPE 7
3	rest	10 min at RPE 6–7; 4 x 2 min at RPE 8 with 2½ min recoveries at RPE 4–5; 10 min at RPE 6–7
4	rest	10 min at RPE 6–7; 5 x 1 min at RPE 8 with 2 min recoveries at RPE 4–5; 10 min at RPE 6–7
5	rest	10 min at RPE 6–7; 20 min at varied pace; 10 min at RPE 6–7
6	rest	10 min at RPE 6–7; 5 x 1½ min at RPE 8 with 2½ min recoveries at RPE 4–5; 10 min at RPE 6–7

WEDNESDAY	THURSDAY	FRIDAY	SATURDAY	SUNDAY
30 min slow at RPE 5–6	10 min at RPE 6–7; 10 min speed or inclines at RPE 8; 10 min at RPE 6–7	rest	40 min at RPE 6	55 min steady at RPE 6–7
30 min at RPE 6	10 min at RPE 6; 15 min speed or inclines at RPE 8; 10 min at RPE 6	rest	40 min at RPE 6	1 hr steady at RPE 6–7
30 min at RPE 6–7	10 min at RPE 6–7; 15 min speed or inclines at RPE 8; 10 min at RPE 6–7	rest	40 min steady at RPE 6–7	1 hr steady at RPE 7

how's it going? ◀◀

WEDNESDAY	THURSDAY	FRIDAY	SATURDAY	SUNDAY
30 min at RPE 7	10 min at RPE 6; stop and stretch, then 1 measured mile (1.5 km) 5 min at RPE 6	rest	40 min steady at RPE 7	1 hr steady at RPE 7–8
30 min at RPE 7–8	10 min at RPE 6–7; 20 min inclines at RPE 8; 10 min at RPE 6–7	rest	30 min steady at RPE 7	45 min slow at RPE 6
rest	10 min at RPE 6–7; 25 min inclines at RPE 8; 10 min at RPE 6–7	rest	30 min slow at RPE 6–7	3 miles (4.8 km)

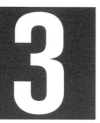

refresher level 4 weeks, repeatable

Level 3, which should be repeated over four weeks, is for those who have had a break in their program or who are walking for at least 12 miles (19.3 km) a week. Use this schedule to train for: improvements in fitness (using four-week training cycles); the first 6-mile (9.6-km) freestyle walk; or a trek/walk for two to three hours with short stops. The mileage starts to creep up at this point and you will cope with this better if you have maintained the previous levels long enough to build a good foundation. Never hesitate to go back a couple of weeks in the schedules if you need to—you will avoid injury.

climbing precautions

Up: Treat a hill like a flight of stairs and take short steps lifting the knees as

level 3 fitness schedule

You need to be able to walk for 45 minutes at a minimum of 3$\frac{1}{2}$ mph (5.6 km/h) for at least 4 days a week before you start this schedule. The fitness schedules will stand you in good stead, either as a basis for moving on to the event schedules, or to repeat (adding in the variations) until you feel comfortable moving on. If the exact day doesn't suit you, because of work or home commitments or because you are tired after the last session, then move the schedules around. Try not to have a break of more than 2 days and remember that a slower or shorter session is better than nothing at all.

WEEK	MONDAY	TUESDAY	
1	rest	10 min slow at RPE 5; 3 x 2 min at RPE 8 with 2 min recoveries at RPE 4–5; 10 min at RPE 6–7	
CYCLE 2		add 1 repeat	
2	rest	10 min steady at RPE 6; 20 min at varied pace; 10 min at RPE 6–7	
CYCLE 2		add 5 min	
3	rest	10 min slow at RPE 5; 4 x 2 min at RPE 8 with 2 min recoveries at RPE 4–5; 10 min at RPE 6–7	
CYCLE 2		add 1 repeat	
4	rest	10 min steady at RPE 6; 2 x 5 min at RPE 8 with 3 min recoveries at RPE 4–5; 4 min at RPE 7	
CYCLE 2		add 1 repeat	

though you have to clear the step. Find a firm footing before you transfer your weight. Lean forward slightly.

Down: Don't come down too fast, and use a goat-like zigzag technique for steep hills. Lean back slightly.

Walking poles and canes are great for giving extra stability on uneven ground. Make sure the pole is adjusted for your height (see pp. 26–27) and use the straps.

week 4—how's it going?

Feeling good? Great, but remember that you are still improving your fitness with shorter or slower walks while you recover from the more intense sessions. So be patient—you can't rush the body. If you are taking longer than a day to recover, then don't push yourself and don't ignore any persistent pains. At the end of week 4, you are ready to start the second cycle, as long as you have had no problems, or alternatively repeat this cycle for as long as you like. Level 4 is the next stage if you are aiming for a race or longer distance.

WEDNESDAY	THURSDAY	FRIDAY	SATURDAY	SUNDAY
35 min at RPE 6–7	10 min slow at RPE 5–6; 5 min brisk at RPE 7–8; 10 min slow at RPE 5–6	rest or 30 min slow	30 min at RPE 6–7	35–45 min steady at RPE 6–7
	add 5 min			add 10 min
35 min at RPE 6	10 min slow at RPE 6; 5 min brisk at RPE 7–8; 10 min slow at RPE 6	rest or 30 min slow	35 min at RPE 6	45–55 min steady at RPE 6–7
	add 5 min			add 10 min
35 min at RPE 6	10 min at RPE 6–7; 5 min at RPE 7–8; 10 min at RPE 6–7	rest or 30 min slow	35 min at RPE 6	50–60 min steady at RPE 6–7
	add 5 min			add 15 min
35 min at RPE 6	10 min at RPE 6; 10 min at RPE 7–8; 10 min at RPE 6	rest	35 min at RPE 6	1 hr–1 hr 10 min steady at RPE 6–7
	add 5 min			add 15 min

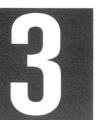

refresher level 6 miles (9.6 km)

You should be able to walk 15 miles (24 km) a week over four or five days before you attempt this schedule. The rate of perceived exertion (RPE) on a scale of 1–10 is shown in each case, indicating workload.

WEEK	MONDAY	TUESDAY	
1	30 min at RPE 6–7 or rest	20 min at RPE 6–7; 4 x 2 min at RPE 8–9 with 2 min recoveries at RPE 4–5; 20 min at RPE 6–7	
2	30 min at RPE 6–7 or rest	20 min at RPE 6–7; 4 x 3 min at RPE 8–9 with 2½ min recoveries at RPE 4–5; 20 min at RPE 6–7	
3	30 min at RPE 6–7 or rest	10 min at RPE 6; stop and stretch, then 2 miles (3 km) 5 min at RPE 6	
4	30 min at RPE 6–7 or rest	20 min at RPE 6–7; 6 x 2 min at RPE 8–9 with 2 min recoveries at RPE 4–5; 20 min at RPE 6–7	
5	30 min at RPE 7 or rest	20 min at RPE 6–7; 5 x 3 min at RPE 8–9 with 2½ min recoveries at RPE 4–5; 20 min at RPE 6–7	
6	30 min at RPE 7	45 min at RPE 7	
7	30 min at RPE 7	45 min at RPE 7–8	
8	rest	cross train 30–60 min	

week 3—how's it going?

You can get an idea of your 6-mile (9.6-km) time from your 1-mile time trial:

MPH	MIN PER MILE	6 MILES (9.6 KM)
3¼	18	1 hr 51 min
3½	17	1 hr 45 min
3¾	16	1 hr 39 min
4	15	1 hr 33 min
4¼	14	1 hr 26 min
4½	13	1 hr 20 min
5	12	1 hr 14 min

You will probably have found your natural pace by now. If you walk faster than 4 miles (6.4 km) per hour, you may find some of the proposed distances less challenging. If that is the case, you may wish to progress more quickly to level 4. Remember to allow the body time to adapt: just because you can walk faster, it doesn't mean you are fit enough to walk long distances yet.

week 6—how's it going?

Keep up the good work: you should be noticing the difference in your fitness and really getting into your stride as soon as you are out the door. If you have a week where you seem to plateau and your fitness doesn't improve, don't worry—improvements are not always visible, but the body is constantly adapting.

WEDNESDAY	THURSDAY	FRIDAY	SATURDAY	SUNDAY
2 miles (3.2 km) at RPE 6–7	10 min at RPE 5–6; 20 min incline at RPE 7–8; 10 min at RPE 5–6	rest	2 miles (3.2 km) at RPE 6–7	3½ miles (5.6 km)
2 miles (3.2 km) at RPE 7–8	20 min at RPE 6; 8 x 1 min hill climb at RPE 8–9 and equal downhill recoveries; 20 min at RPE 6	rest	walk/cross train 30–60 min	4 miles (6.5 km)
2½ miles (4 km) at RPE 6–7	10 min at RPE 5–6; 30 min inclines up and down at RPE 7–8; 10 min at RPE 5–6	rest	3 miles (4.8 km) at RPE 7	4½ miles (7 km)

◀◀ how's it going?

2½ miles (4 km) at RPE 7–8	20 min at RPE 6; 10 x 1 min hill climb at RPE 8–9 and equal downhill recoveries; 20 min at RPE 6	rest	3½ miles (5.6 km) at RPE 6–7	5 miles (8 km)
3 miles (4.8 km) at RPE 6–7	10 min at RPE 5–6; 40 min incline at RPE 7–8; 10 min at RPE 5–6	rest	walk /cross train 30–60 min	5½ miles (8.5 km)
3 miles (4.8 km) at RPE 7	20 min at RPE 6; 12 x 1 min hill climb at RPE 8–9 and equal downhill recoveries; 20 min at RPE 6	rest	3½ miles (5.6 km) at RPE 7	6 miles (9.6 km)

▲ how's it going?

3 miles (4.8 km) at RPE 7–8	20 min at RPE 6; 8 x 2 min hill climb at RPE 9 and equal downhill recoveries; 20 min at RPE 6	rest	4 miles (6.5 km) at RPE 6–7	4 miles (6.5 km)
3½ miles (5.6 km) at RPE 6–7	rest or slow 30 min	rest	2 miles (3 km) at RPE 6	6 miles (9.6 km) in under 2 hours

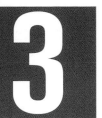

refresher level 3-hour trek

Follow this schedule over a six-week period and see if you can complete a half-day trek in three hours. Be careful while out on the route.

don't get lost, don't panic

The key to this schedule is to get used to walking while following a map or route markers. You need to have confidence that you are going the right way (it may feel like a long time before the next marker), and pick up signs that you are still on track along the route. If you do make a mistake, you may be able to find another way around, or you may have to retrace your steps. Don't forget to take a compass—it may save you time if you lose your way.

You can avoid getting lost by:
- going with someone who knows the route well
- following a well-marked route
- sticking to paths and well-used routes, where you may meet other walkers
- using a map and compass.

If you do get lost, don't panic. Try to establish where you are by looking for landmarks that you can match to your map. Call and let someone know you may be longer than planned, and decide whether to try to make your way to another part of the planned route or retrace your steps. If it is likely to get dark before you get back, be cautious, and choose the shortest return route.

WEEK	MONDAY	TUESDAY	WEDNESDAY
1	rest	2 miles (3.2 km) at RPE 7 (timed)	off road over different terrains; 30 min at RPE 6
2	rest	cross train 30–60 min	off road over different terrains; 30 min at RPE 6–7
3	rest	2 miles (3.2 km) at RPE 7 (timed)	off road over different terrains; 30 min at RPE 7
4	rest	cross train 30–60 min	off road over different terrains; 45 min at RPE 6
5	rest	2 miles (3.2 km) at RPE 7 (timed)	off road over different terrains; 45 min at RPE 6–7
6	rest	cross train 30–60 min	20 min at RPE 6; 12 x 1 min steep hill climb at RPE 8–9 and downhill recoveries; 20 min at RPE 6

week 3—how's it going?

Try to stick to the schedule—it is demanding but it will provide a solid foundation for the next stage, the intermediate level. However, don't move on until you feel you are ready.

THURSDAY	FRIDAY	SATURDAY	SUNDAY
on road or grass; 45 min at RPE 6	10 min at RPE 5–6; 20 min incline at RPE 7–8; 10 min at RPE 5–6	30 min at RPE 6–7	1 hr walk
on road or grass; 45 min at RPE 6–7	20 min at RPE 6; 8 x 1 min steep hill climb at RPE 8–9 and downhill recoveries; 20 min at RPE 6	30 min at RPE 7	1 hr 15 min over natural terrains and inclines
on road or grass; 50 min at RPE 6–7	10 min at RPE 5–6; 30 min incline at RPE 7–8; 10 min at RPE 5–6	30 min at RPE 7–8	1 1/2 hr walk

≜ how's it going?

on road or grass; 55 min at RPE 6–7	20 min at RPE 6; 10 x 1 min steep hill climb at RPE 8–9 and downhill recoveries; 20 min at RPE 6	45 min at RPE 6–7	2 hr walk with short stops
on road or grass; 1 hr at RPE 6	10 min at RPE 5–6; 40 min incline at RPE 7–8; 10 min at RPE 5–6	45 min at RPE 7	1 1/2 hr walk
rest	off road over different terrains; 45 min at RPE 7	rest	**half-day trek** 9–12 miles (14.5–19 km)

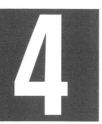

intermediate level

You are ready for this level if you are walking four days a week and a total distance of 16–20 miles (26–32 km) a week. You should be able to walk 3 miles (4.8 km) easily in less than an hour. The aim of this schedule is to build up time spent on your feet and this program will also provide a good start for those who wish to train for a marathon. There is a schedule for a fitness program (4-week training cycles), a walk of more than 10 miles (16 plus km) in about three hours on flat terrain, a 6-mile (9.6-km) event walk and a five- to seven-hour trek over natural terrain. (If you plan to do the event walk, see pp. 50–51 on event walking rules.)

interval guide (speed work)

No matter how fast you can go, you need more than just your legs to walk fast for any distance. The strength and stamina of your heart, lungs, and upper body also dictate how long you can keep it up. Over a distance of 5 miles (8 km) you should aim to spend at least 5 minutes of every mile or kilometer walking at speed (intervals) or up and down hills.

WEEK	MONDAY	TUESDAY
1	rest	10 min slow at RPE 5; 5 x 2 min at RPE 8 with 2 min recoveries at RPE 4–5; 10 min at RPE 6–7
CYCLE **2**		add 1 repeat
2	rest	10 min steady at RPE 6; 30 min varied pace; 10 min at RPE 6–7
CYCLE **2**		add 5 min
3	rest	10 min slow at RPE 5; 6 x 2 min at RPE 8 with 2 min recoveries at RPE 4–5; 10 min at RPE 6–7
CYCLE **2**		add 1 repeat
4	rest	10 min steady at RPE 6; 3 x 5 min at RPE 8 with 3 min recoveries at RPE 4–5; 4 min at RPE 7
CYCLE **2**		add 1 repeat

If you are working through the levels, you will be equipped to start this level, but if your usual distance is only 16 miles (25.7 km) a week, then keep to the fitness schedules for four more weeks before starting on the events. You can then add in the variations in the second cycle as you work toward the race schedules.

week 4—how's it going?

You have done really well to get here, so congratulate yourself. But if you are very tired for the rest of the day after your walks or you are suffering from persistent pains, then you could take it a bit easier. Replace the harder or longer walks with an easy day, or rest completely. You are aiming for a regular walking schedule, and you can still improve your fitness with shorter or slower walks while you recover from the more intense sessions. At the end of week 4, you are ready to start the second cycle, as long as you have had no problems, or alternatively repeat this cycle for as long as you like. Move up to level 5 when you feel ready.

	WEDNESDAY	THURSDAY		FRIDAY	SATURDAY	SUNDAY
	35 min at RPE 6–7	10 min slow at RPE 5–6; 15 min brisk at RPE 7–8; 10 min slow at RPE 5–6		rest or 30 min slow	30 min at RPE 6–7	30–45 min steady at RPE 6–7
		add 5 min				add 10 min
	35 min at RPE 6	10 min slow at RPE 6; 15 min brisk at RPE 7–8; 10 min slow at RPE 6		rest or 30 min slow	40 min at RPE 6	45–60 min steady at RPE 6–7
		add 5 min				add 15 min
	35 min at RPE 6	10 min at RPE 6–7; 20 min at RPE 7–8; 10 min at RPE 6–7		rest or 30 min slow	40 min at RPE 6	50–70 min steady at RPE 6–7
		add 5 min				add 15 min
	35 min at RPE 6	10 min at RPE 6; 20 min at RPE 7–8; 10 min at RPE 6		rest	40 min at RPE 6	60–90 min steady at RPE 6–7
		add 5 min				add 20 min

4

intermediate level 6 miles (9.6 km)

If your measured time trial came out at more than 30 minutes (4 mph [6.4 km/h]), then stick with the schedules. Then when you set off on the race at your target pace, speed up only when you pass the halfway marker if it feels comfortable. If your pace is faster than 4 mph (6.4 km/h), walk at a slightly slower pace every 10 minutes during the race to give your hips a change of position and to help you maintain your energy throughout the event.

WEEK	MONDAY	TUESDAY	WEDNESDAY	
1	30 min at RPE 6–7 or rest	20 min at RPE 6–7; 4 x 2 min at RPE 8–9 with 2 min recoveries at RPE 4–5; 20 min at RPE 6–7	2 miles (3.2 km) at RPE 6–7	
2	30 min at RPE 6–7 or rest	20 min at RPE 6–7; 4 x 3 min at RPE 8–9 with 2½ min recoveries at RPE 4–5; 20 min at RPE 6–7	2 miles (3.2 km) at RPE 7–8	
3	30 min at RPE 6–7 or rest	10 min at RPE 6; stop and stretch, then 2 miles (3 km) 5 min at RPE 6	2½ miles (4 km) at RPE 6–7	
4	30 min at RPE 6–7 or rest	20 min at RPE 6–7; 6 x 2 min at RPE 8–9 with 2 min recoveries at RPE 4–5; 20 min at RPE 6–7	2½ miles (4 km) at RPE 7–8	
5	30 min at RPE 7 or rest	20 min at RPE 6–7; 5 x 3 min at RPE 8–9 with 2½ min recoveries at RPE 4–5; 20 min at RPE 6–7	3 miles (4.8 km) at RPE 6–7	
6	30 min at RPE 7	45 min at RPE 7	3 miles (4.8 km) at RPE 7	
7	30 min at RPE 7	45 min at RPE 7–8	3 miles (4.8 km) at RPE 7–8	
8	rest	cross train 30–60 min	3½ miles (5.6 km) at RPE 6–7	

THURSDAY	FRIDAY	SATURDAY	SUNDAY
10 min at RPE 5–6; 20 min incline at RPE 7–8; 10 min at RPE 5–6	rest	2 miles (3.2 km) at RPE 6–7	3½ miles (5.6 km)
20 min at RPE 6; 8 x 1 min hill climb at RPE 8–9 and equal downhill recoveries; 20 min at RPE 6	rest	walk or cross train 30–60 min	4½ miles (7 km)
10 min at RPE 5–6; 30 min inclines up and down at RPE 7–8; 10 min at RPE 5–6	rest	3 miles (4.8 km) at RPE 7	5½ miles (8.5 km)
20 min at RPE 6; 10 x 1 min hill climb at RPE 8–9 and equal downhill recoveries; 20 min at RPE 6	rest	3½ miles (5.6 km) at RPE 6–7	7 miles (11 km)
10 min at RPE 5–6; 40 min incline at RPE 7–8; 10 min at RPE 5–6	rest	walk or cross train 30–60 min	7½ miles (12 km)
20 min at RPE 6; 12 x 1 min hill climb at RPE 8–9 and equal downhill recoveries; 20 min at RPE 6	rest	3½ miles (5.6 km) at RPE 7	8½ miles (13.5 km)
20 min at RPE 6; 8 x 2 min hill climb at RPE 9 and equal downhill recoveries; 20 min at RPE 6	rest	4 miles (6.5 km) at RPE 6–7	4 miles (6.5 km)
rest or slow 30 min	rest	2 miles (3.2 km) at RPE 6	6 miles (9.6 km) in 2 hr

HOW LONG WILL IT TAKE?

If you want to know how long it will take to walk 10 miles, 10 kilometers, or any other distance in a 4-hour trek (you have to allow for uneven terrain, so the pace will be slightly slower) you can get a rough idea from a measured time trial. Walk at a comfortable, brisk pace for a measured distance of 2 miles (3.2 km).

MPH	MIN PER MILE	6 MILES (9.6 KM)	10 MILES (16 KM)
3	20	2 hr	3 hr 20 min
3¼	18	1 hr 51 min	3 hr 5 min
3½	17	1 hr 43 min	2 hr 51 min
3¾	16	1 hr 36 min	2 hr 40 min
4	15	1 hr 30 min	2 hr 30 min
4¼	14	1 hr 25 min	2 hr 21 min
4½	13	1 hr 20 min	2 hr 13 min
5	12	1 hr 12 min	2 hr

10-MILE (16-KM) FLAT WALK

Aim for a walk that lasts between two and three hours. The trick is to pace yourself so that the last mile feels almost as good as the first. Your legs will be tired, but if you build up your pace steadily in the first few miles, 10 miles (16 km) will feel like half the distance. Unless you have good reason to stop, keep moving all the time, slowing down a little while you eat or drink.

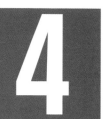

intermediate day-long trek

I f possible, do the Sunday walk on surfaces and gradients that will be similar (slightly less demanding) to those walked during the planned event day.

day-trek schedule

(5-7 hour walk)
You need to be able to walk for at least 4 hours a week before you start this schedule. You might be able to do it immediately, but a 4-hour trek over rough ground will tax you if you are not prepared. In 4 hours, you could cover 12–18 miles (19–29 km) depending on the terrain and your fitness. Trekking will also often include stops to look at the view, so this gives you a chance to rest.

week 4—how's it going?

The main objectives of this schedule are to build stamina in your legs and to get used to being on your feet (or in your shoes) for hours at a time. It is also a chance to get used to the extra mileage walking with poles or walking canes. Walking poles can involve an extra 25 to 30 percent of extra energy, so you need to get used to using them. Make sure you look after your feet carefully and allow yourself enough time at the weekends to fit in the longer walks.

WEEK	MONDAY	TUESDAY	WEDNESDAY
1	rest	2 miles (3.2 km) at RPE 7 (timed)	off road over different terrains; 30 min at RPE 6
2	rest	cross train 30–60 min	off road over different terrains; 30 min at RPE 6–7
3	rest	2 miles (3.2 km) at RPE 7 (timed)	off road over different terrains; 30 min at RPE 7
4	rest	cross train 30–60 min	off road over different terrains; 45 min at RPE 6
5	rest	2 miles (3.2 km) at RPE 7 (timed)	off road over different terrains; 45 min at RPE 6–7
6	rest	cross train 30–60 min	20 min at RPE 6; 12 x 1 min steep hill climb at RPE 8–9 and downhill recoveries; 20 min at RPE 6

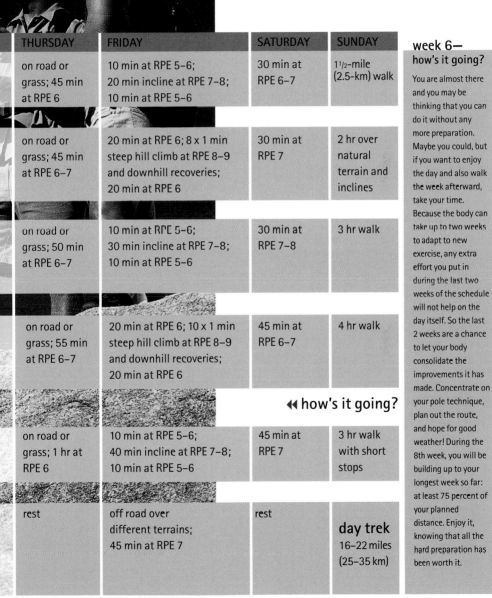

THURSDAY	FRIDAY	SATURDAY	SUNDAY
on road or grass; 45 min at RPE 6	10 min at RPE 5–6; 20 min incline at RPE 7–8; 10 min at RPE 5–6	30 min at RPE 6–7	1½-mile (2.5-km) walk
on road or grass; 45 min at RPE 6–7	20 min at RPE 6; 8 x 1 min steep hill climb at RPE 8–9 and downhill recoveries; 20 min at RPE 6	30 min at RPE 7	2 hr over natural terrain and inclines
on road or grass; 50 min at RPE 6–7	10 min at RPE 5–6; 30 min incline at RPE 7–8; 10 min at RPE 5–6	30 min at RPE 7–8	3 hr walk
on road or grass; 55 min at RPE 6–7	20 min at RPE 6; 10 x 1 min steep hill climb at RPE 8–9 and downhill recoveries; 20 min at RPE 6	45 min at RPE 6–7	4 hr walk
on road or grass; 1 hr at RPE 6	10 min at RPE 5–6; 40 min incline at RPE 7–8; 10 min at RPE 5–6	45 min at RPE 7	3 hr walk with short stops
rest	off road over different terrains; 45 min at RPE 7	rest	**day trek** 16–22 miles (25–35 km)

◀◀ **how's it going?**

week 6— how's it going?

You are almost there and you may be thinking that you can do it without any more preparation. Maybe you could, but if you want to enjoy the day and also walk the week afterward, take your time. Because the body can take up to two weeks to adapt to new exercise, any extra effort you put in during the last two weeks of the schedule will not help on the day itself. So the last 2 weeks are a chance to let your body consolidate the improvements it has made. Concentrate on your pole technique, plan out the route, and hope for good weather! During the 8th week, you will be building up to your longest week so far: at least 75 percent of your planned distance. Enjoy it, knowing that all the hard preparation has been worth it.

how's it going? ▶▶

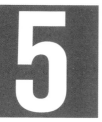

upper level

Level 5 is for those who can walk four to six days a week covering a weekly distance of 20 to 30 miles (32–48 km). It contains a fitness running schedule, a fast 6-mile (9.6-km) event, a half-marathon schedule, and a weekend trek (8–16 hours) over rough terrain. If you want to walk longer rather than train for a specific event, this level is for you. If you are training for the half marathon or the weekend trek, work backward from the proposed date, and plan to start the schedule with about a week to spare.

level 5 fitness schedule

Before you start this schedule, which can be repeated over 4 weeks, you should be able to walk for 45 to 60 minutes 5–6 days a week with regular speed or hill work. Use the fitness schedule by first following the standard sessions. To progress when you have comfortably completed the first 4 weeks, repeat the schedule, adding in the variations in the second cycle. When you are training for longer distances, you can repeat your long Sunday walks on shorter sessions, because the one Sunday walk is meant for those who would not otherwise do a long walk. If you are planning the weekend trek, see the box to the right.

WEEK	MONDAY	TUESDAY
1	rest	10 min steady at RPE 6; 4 x 4 min at RPE 8 with 2 min recoveries at RPE 4–5; 10 min at RPE 6–7
CYCLE 2		add 2 repeats
2	rest	10 min steady at RPE 6; 30 min varied pace; 10 min at RPE 6–7
CYCLE 2		add 5 min
3	rest	10 min steady at RPE 7; 5 x 5 min at RPE 8 with 2 min recoveries at RPE 5 –6; 10 min at RPE 6–7
CYCLE 2		add 2 repeats
4	rest	10 min steady at RPE 6; 6 x 6 min at RPE 8 with 3 min recoveries at RPE 4–5; 4 min at RPE 7
CYCLE 2		add 1 repeat

how do I train for an event that lasts more than a day?

To train the body to work hard, rest, and then work hard immediately, it is important to do a longer stint on both Saturday and Sunday. Normally, you would be advised to have a rest day in between hard sessions. When your body needs to maximize energy stores to repeat the same workout, there are certain strategies that help:

- Keep your energy levels up during the day with carbohydrate-rich foods and energy drinks.
- Get plenty of rest—don't join in intense physical activities on the first evening.
- Eat enough in the evening to replenish your energy stores, but not so much that feeling stuffed prevents you from sleeping.
- If you have strained anything, use ice to reduce the inflammation.
- Make sure that anything you need to carry is packed well, because it will be on your back for a long time.
- If you don't feel well, don't be too proud to say you cannot finish the second day.

WEDNESDAY	THURSDAY	FRIDAY	SATURDAY	SUNDAY
40 min at RPE 6–7	10 min slow at RPE 5–6; 20 min brisk at RPE 7–8; 10 min slow at RPE 5–6	rest or 30 min slow	40 min at RPE 6–7	45–55 min steady at RPE 6–7
	add 5 min			add 10 min
40 min at RPE 6	10 min slow at RPE 6; 20 min brisk at RPE 7–8; 10 min slow at RPE 6	rest or 30 min slow	45 min at RPE 6	55–65 min steady at RPE 6–7
	add 5 min			add 10 min
40 min at RPE 6	10 min at RPE 6–7; 30 min at RPE 7–8; 10 min at RPE 6–7	rest or 30 min slow	45 min at RPE 6	1 hr 10 min– 1 hr 20 min steady at RPE 6–7
	add 5 min			add 15 min
35 min at RPE 6	10 min at RPE 6; 20 min at RPE 7–8; 10 min at RPE 6	rest	45 min at RPE 6	1 hr 30 min –1 hr 40 min steady at RPE 6–7
	add 10 min			add 10 min

week 4— how's it going?

By the end of week 4, if you have no problems, you are ready to start the second cycle or repeat this cycle for as long as you like. Only go on to the next part of the schedule when you feel ready.

5

upper level 6 miles (9.6 km)

WEEK	MONDAY	TUESDAY	WEDNESDAY
1	30 min at RPE 6–7 or rest	20 min at RPE 6–7; 4 x 3 min at RPE 8–9 with 2 min recoveries at RPE 4–5; 20 min at RPE 6–7	2 miles (3.2 km) at RPE 7–8
2	30 min at RPE 6–7 or rest	20 min at RPE 6–7; 4 x 4 min at RPE 8–9 with 2½ min recoveries at RPE 4–5; 20 min at RPE 6–7	2 miles (3.2 km) at RPE 7–8
3	30 min at RPE 6–7 or rest	10 min at RPE 6; stop and stretch, then 2 miles (3 km) 5 min at RPE 6	2½ miles (4 km) at RPE 6–7
4	30 min at RPE 6–7 or rest	20 min at RPE 6–7; 6 x 3 min at RPE 8–9 with 2 min recoveries at RPE 4–5; 20 min at RPE 6–7	2½ miles (4 km) at RPE 7–8
5	30 min at RPE 7 or rest	20 min at RPE 6–7; 5 x 4 min at RPE 8–9 with 2.5 min recoveries at RPE 4–5; 20 min at RPE 6–7	3 miles (4.8 km) at RPE 6–7
6	30 min at RPE 7	45 min at RPE 8	3 miles (4.8 km) at RPE 7
7	30 min at RPE 7	45 min at RPE 7–8	3 miles (4.8 km) at RPE 7–8
8	rest	cross train 30–60 min	3½ miles (5.6 km) at RPE 7–8

Before you begin this schedule, you should be walking 6 days a week and covering at least 20 miles (32 km).

event walking
This schedule is to get you up to speed. Competitive event power walkers can walk 1 mile (1.5 km) in less than 10 minutes, but this level of experience can take years to achieve. If participating in this type of event is your goal, join a club. They can advise you on technique and race know-how, and it also gives you the chance to train with other people.

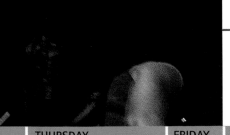

THURSDAY	FRIDAY	SATURDAY	SUNDAY
10 min at RPE 5–6; 20 min incline at RPE 7–8; 10 min at RPE 5–6	rest	4 miles (6.5 km) at RPE 6–7	5 miles (8 km)
20 min at RPE 6; 8 x 1 min hill climb at RPE 8–9 and equal downhill recoveries; 20 min at RPE 6	rest	walk or cross train 30–60 min	3 miles (4.8 km) fast at RPE 8
10 min at RPE 5–6; 30 min incline up and down RPE 7–8; 10 min at RPE 5–6	rest	3 miles (4.8 km) at RPE 7	4 1/2 miles (7 km)
20 min at RPE 6; 10 x 1 min hill climb at RPE 8–9 and equal downhill recoveries; 20 min at RPE 6	rest	3 1/2 miles (5.6 km) at RPE 6–7	5 miles (8 km)
10 min at RPE 5–6; 40 min incline at RPE 7–8; 10 min at RPE 5–6	rest	walk or cross train 30–60 min	5 1/2 miles (8.5 km)
20 min at RPE 6; 12 x 1 min hill climb at RPE 8–9 and equal downhill recoveries; 20 min at RPE 6	rest	3 1/2 miles (5.6 km) at RPE 7	6 miles (9.6 km)
20 min at RPE 6; 8 x 2 min hill climb at RPE 9 and equal downhill recoveries; 20 min at RPE 6	rest	4 miles (6.5 km) at RPE 6–7	4 miles (6.5 km)
rest or slow 30 min	rest	2 miles (3.2 km) at RPE 6	6 miles (9.6 km) in less than 1 hr 30 min

how's it going?

week 4
work out your 6-mile (9.6-km) target time from the 1-mile (1.5- km) time trial.

16 min a mile = 1 hr 39 min

15 min a mile = 1 hr 33 min

14 min a mile = 1 hr 26 min

13 min a mile = 1 hr 20 min

12 min a mile = 1 hr 14 min

week 6
half-marathon times
The 6-mile (9.6-km) walk on Sunday will indicate your expected time for a half-marathon (13 miles [20.9 km]). You may need to add 5 to 10 percent of the predicted time to allow for drink stops, change of pace, or slower walking—all important allowances during a longer walk.

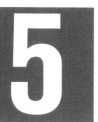

upper level half-marathon

This schedule assumes a weekly mileage of 25 miles (40 km), with two two-hour walks at the weekend.

speed or strength?

Speed is not of the essence for this schedule: strength and stamina are.

WEEK	MONDAY	TUESDAY	WEDNESDAY	
1	rest	15 min at RPE 6–7; 4 x 2 min at RPE 8–9 with 2 min recoveries at RPE 4–5; 15 min at RPE 6–7	2 miles (3.2 km) at RPE 6–7	
2	rest	15 min at RPE 6–7; 4 x 3 min at RPE 8–9 with 2½ min recoveries at RPE 4–5; 15 min at RPE 6–7	cross train 30–60 min	
3	rest	15 min at RPE 6–7; 6 x 2 min at RPE 8–9 with 2 min recoveries at RPE 4–5; 15 min at RPE 6–7	3½ miles (5.6 km) at RPE 6–7	
4	rest	15 min at RPE 6–7; 5 x 3 min at RPE 8–9 with 2 ½ min recoveries at RPE 4–5; 15 min at RPE 6–7	cross train 30–60 min	
5	rest	15 min at RPE 6–7; 6 x 2 min at RPE 8–9 with 2 min recoveries at RPE 4–5; 15 min at RPE 6–7	4 miles (6.5 km) at RPE 6–7	
6	rest	1 hr at RPE 7–8	3 miles (4.8 km) at RPE 6–7	
7	rest	15 min at RPE 6–7; 6 x 3 min at RPE 8–9 with 2½ min recoveries at RPE 4–5; 15 min at RPE 6–7	cross train 30–60 min	
8	rest	45 min at RPE 7–8	4 miles (6.5 km) at RPE 6–7	
9	rest	45 min at RPE 7– 8	5 miles (8 km) at RPE 6–7	
10	rest	30 min at RPE 7	rest	

week 4— how's it going?

Knowing that you can stop during the day should overcome any doubts you have about your ability to keep up with everyone else. However, you want to enjoy the weekend and not end up stiff and sore. You have gotten this far, so there shouldn't be any problems if you keep to the schedule. However, don't ignore any pains just because you are so close to your goal. There is time enough to get them sorted out and you will still be able to walk. If you leave it much longer, it may stop you completely. Don't risk it.

However, don't forget that hill work is comparable to speed work, so if you can't find any hills to walk, slip in an interval session instead. You need to build up time on your feet but you also need to get used to carrying a pack on your back. Use the longer sessions to acclimatize yourself to the extra weight: it will also make you think twice about what you really need.

THURSDAY	FRIDAY	SATURDAY	SUNDAY
10 min at RPE 5–6; 20 min inclines at RPE 7–8; 10 min at RPE 5–6	off road; 2 miles (3.2 km) at RPE 6–7	30 min at RPE 6–7	4 miles (6.5 km)
20 min at RPE 6; 8 x 1 min steep hill climb at RPE 8–9 and downhill recoveries; 20 min at RPE 6	off road; 2 miles (3.2 km) at RPE 7–8	30 min at RPE 6–7	5 miles (8 km)
20 min at RPE 6; 10 x 1 min steep hill climb at RPE 8–9 and downhill recoveries; 20 min at RPE 6	off road; 2½ miles (4 km) at RPE 7–8	35 min at RPE 6–7	6 miles (9.6 km)
10 min at RPE 5–6; 40 min incline at RPE 7–8; 10 min at RPE 5–6	off road; 3 miles (4.8 km) at RPE 6–7	40 min at RPE 6–7	7 miles (11 km)

◄◄ how's it going?

THURSDAY	FRIDAY	SATURDAY	SUNDAY
20 min at RPE 6; 8 x 2 min steep hill climb at RPE 9 and downhill recoveries; 20 min at RPE 6	off road; 3 miles (4.8 km) at RPE 7–8	45 min at RPE 6–7	8 miles (13 km)
20 min at RPE 6; 10 x 2 min steep hill climb at RPE 8–9 and downhill recoveries; 20 min at RPE 6	off road; 3½ miles (5.6 km) at RPE 7–8	1 hr at RPE 6–7	9 miles (14.5 km)
20 min at RPE 6; 12 x 2 min steep hill climb at RPE 8–9 and downhill recoveries; 20 min at RPE 6	off road; 4 miles (6.5 km) at RPE 7–8	1 hr at RPE 6–7	10 miles (16 km)
30 min inclines at RPE 7	cross train 30–60 min	45 min at RPE 6–7	11 miles (17.5 km)

how's it going? ►►

THURSDAY	FRIDAY	SATURDAY	SUNDAY
30 min inclines at RPE 7	3½ miles (5.6 km) at RPE 6–7	30 min at RPE 6–7	6 miles (9.6 km)
30 min at RPE 6–7	cross train 30–60 min or slow walk	rest	half-marathon

week 8—
how's it going?

The last 2 weeks should be spent concentrating on making sure everything is in place: travel and accommodation are organized, rest or water stops are planned if necessary, and anything you need has been bought and packed. Your training should be tapering down over the next 2 weeks to leave you plenty of energy for the day.

5 upper level weekend trek

The Sunday walk is to be undertaken over surfaces and gradients that will be similar (slightly less demanding) than those walked during the trek.

orienteering

If you want to try something a bit different, try some orienteering. This is not just about fitness or speed but will also test your initiative and navigation skills. Working out the shortest route, identifying the route markers, and working alone or with others are all part of the challenge.

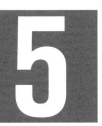

WEEK	MONDAY	TUESDAY	WEDNESDAY
1	rest	2 miles (3.2 km) at RPE 7	off road over different terrains; 30 min at RPE 6
2	rest	cross train 30–60 min	off road over different terrains; 30 min at RPE 6–7
3	rest	2 miles (3.2 km) at RPE 7	off road over different terrains; 30 min at RPE 7
4	rest	cross train 30–60 min	off road over different terrains; 45 min at RPE 6
5	rest	2 miles (3.2 km) at RPE 7	off road over different terrains; 45 min at RPE 6–7
6	rest	cross train 30–60 min	off road over different terrains; 45 min at RPE 7
7	rest	3 miles (4.8 km) at RPE 7–8	off road over different terrains; 45 min at RPE 7
8	rest	cross train 30–60 min	rest

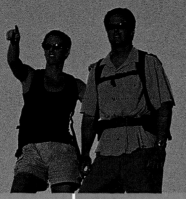

THURSDAY	FRIDAY	SATURDAY	SUNDAY
on road or grass; 45 min at RPE 6	10 min at RPE 5–6; 20 min incline at RPE 7–8; 10 min at RPE 5–6	1 hr at RPE 6–7	1 hr walk
on road or grass; 45 min at RPE 6–7	20 min at RPE 6; 8 x 1 min steep hill climb at RPE 8–9 and downhill recoveries; 20 min at RPE 6	1½ hr at RPE 7	5 miles (8 km) over terrain and inclines 2 hr walk
on road or grass; 50 min at RPE 6–7	10 min at RPE 5–6; 30 min incline at RPE 7–8; 10 min at RPE 5–6	2 hr at RPE 7–8	3 hr walk
on road or grass; 55 min at RPE 6–7	20 min at RPE 6; 10 x 1 min steep hill climb at RPE 8–9 and downhill recoveries; 20 min at RPE 6	3 hr at RPE 6–7	4 hr walk
on road or grass; 1 hr at RPE 6–7	10 min at RPE 5–6; 40 min incline at RPE 7–8; 10 min at RPE 5–6	4 hr at RPE 7	4 hr walk
on road or grass; 1 hr at RPE 6–7	20 min at RPE 6; 12 x 1 min steep hill climb at RPE 8–9 and downhill recoveries; 20 min at RPE 6	5 hr walk	5 hr walk
on road or grass; 1 hr at RPE 6–7	rest	1½ hr at RPE 7	2 hr walk with short stops
on road or grass; 1 hr at RPE 6–7	rest	**weekend trek** 20 plus miles (32 plus km)	

6 advanced level

This final level is for walkers who spend at least one day a week walking for two hours and four days a week for one hour at about 4 mph (6.4 km/h). In this schedule, you will find a program for fitness (with four-week training cycles), a charity event marathon, a marathon event walk, and a weeklong trekking expedition. Do not sacrifice speed sessions for distance or think

level 6 fitness schedules

You need to be able to walk on most days of the week and cover at least 24 miles (38.6 km) a week. This fitness schedule includes the main sessions, with the variations added in after 4 weeks. Like the other schedules, it is repeatable on other weeks, or it can be a launch pad for the next parts of the schedule. Follow the schedule to your goal and return to this foundation if you need to take off more than a week from the target schedule.

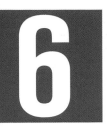

WEEK	MONDAY	TUESDAY
1	rest	10 min steady at RPE 6; 5 x 4 min at RPE 8 with 2 min recoveries at RPE 4–5; 10 min at RPE 6–7
CYCLE 2		add 2 repeats
2	rest	10 min steady at RPE 6; 30 min varied pace; 10 min at RPE 6–7
CYCLE 2		add 10 min
3	rest	10 min steady at RPE 7; 7 x 4 min at RPE 8 with 2 min recoveries at RPE 4–5; 10 min at RPE 6–7
CYCLE 2		add 3 repeats
4	rest	10 min steady at RPE 6; 5 x 5 min at RPE 8 with 3 min recoveries at RPE 4–5; 4 min at RPE 7
CYCLE 2		add 2 repeats

that distance alone will be enough: you need all aspects of the training schedule, even more so for this final level, to know that you are getting the best for all your hard work.

cross training

Many walkers feel that they don't need to do anything other than walking to maintain fitness. Although this is true up to a point, if you are recovering from an injury or the weather is bad, the gym or swimming pool offer alternatives that will help you to train just as effectively. Even minor irritations such as blisters that may stop you from walking should not stop you from using weight-training machines, a bicycle, a rowing machine, or a swimming pool.

WEDNESDAY	THURSDAY	FRIDAY	SATURDAY	SUNDAY
35 min at RPE 6–7	10 min slow at RPE 5–6; 20 min brisk RPE 7–8; 10 min slow at RPE 5–6	rest or 30 min slow	40 min at RPE 6–7	45–60 min steady at RPE 6–7
	add 10 min			add 15 min
35 min at RPE 6	10 min slow at RPE 6; 20 min brisk RPE 7–8; 10 min slow at RPE 6	rest or 30 min slow	45 min at RPE 6	1–1 1/2 hr steady at RPE 6–7
	add 10 min			add 15 min
35 min at RPE 6	10 min at RPE 6–7; 30 min RPE 7–8; 10 min at RPE 6–7	rest or 30 min slow	45 min at RPE 6	1 1/2–2 hr steady at RPE 6–7
	add 10 min			add 20 min
35 min at RPE 6	10 min at RPE 6; 20 min RPE 7–8; 10 min at RPE 6	rest	45 min at RPE 6	1 1/2–2 hr steady at RPE 6–7
	add 5 min			add 15 min

week 4— how's it going?

Whichever goal you are aiming for, you now need to build up your distance and stay injury-free. Consider having a monthly massage, or visit a sports therapist to check that you are not building up any physical problems for the future. Progress to the second cycle as a precursor to the final part of the schedules.

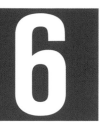

advanced level marathon walk

(the Sunday walk should be on similar surfaces to those predicted for the marathon)

The experience of participating in a marathon is always a personally rewarding one, although people take part for different reasons—for fun, for charity, or simply for the challenge of competing with other contenders. Whatever your motivation, the buildup on the day is exhilarating. Public

week 8— how's it going?

You should be increasing your long walks by 1-2 miles (1.5-3 km) a week so that you reach the target test walk with 2 weeks to spare. You are halfway there now and this last 8 weeks is the time to relish your achievements so far. If you are collecting for charity, talk to all your friends and family: you can be pretty sure that, failing injury, you will be able to do it, no matter how unlikely it might have seemed when you first signed up.

WEEK	MONDAY	TUESDAY	WEDNESDAY	
1	30 min at RPE 6–7	15 min at RPE 6–7; 2 x 4 min at RPE 8–9 with 2 min recoveries at RPE 4–5; 15 min at RPE 6–7	2 miles (3.2 km) at RPE 6–7	
2	30 min at RPE 6–7	15 min at RPE 6–7; 2 x 6 min at RPE 8–9 with 4 min recoveries at RPE 4–5; 15 min at RPE 6–7	2 miles (3.2 km) at RPE 7–8	
3	30 min at RPE 6–7	15 min at RPE 6–7; 4, 6, 4 min at RPE 8–9 with 4 min recoveries at RPE 4–5; 15 min at RPE 6–7	2¹/₂ miles (4 km) at RPE 6–7	
4	35 min at RPE 6–7	15 min at RPE 6–7; 6 x 2 min at RPE 8–9 with 2 min recoveries at RPE 4–5; 15 min at RPE 6–7	2¹/₂ miles (4 km) at RPE 7–8	
5	40 min at RPE 6–7	15 min at RPE 6–7; 3 x 4 min at RPE 8–9 with 2 min recoveries at RPE 4–5; 15 min at RPE 6–7	3 miles (4.8 km) at RPE 6–7	
6	45 min at RPE 6–7	10 min at RPE 6–7; 3 x 6 min at RPE 8–9 with 4 min recoveries at RPE 4–5; 10 min at RPE 6–7	3 miles (4.8 km) at RPE 7–8	
7	45 min at RPE 6–7	10 min at RPE 6–7; 6, 4, 2, 4, 6 min at RPE 8–9 with half as long recoveries at RPE 4–5; 10 min at RPE 6–7	3 miles (4.8 km) at RPE 7–8	
8	45 min at RPE 6–7	15 min at RPE 6–7; 8 x 2 min at RPE 8–9 with 2 min recoveries at RPE 4–5; 15 min at RPE 6–7	3¹/₂ miles (5.6 km) at RPE 6–7	

transportation (sometimes free to participants) is packed with walkers or runners, and events are usually well run with a lively atmosphere.

THURSDAY	FRIDAY	SATURDAY	SUNDAY
off road; 2 1/2 miles (4 km)	rest	45 min at RPE 5–6	5 1/2 miles (8.5 km)
10 min at RPE 5–6; 20 min incline at RPE 7–8; 10 min at RPE 5–6	rest	cross train 30–60 min	6 1/2 miles (10.5 km)
20 min at RPE 6; 8 x 1 min steep hill climb at RPE 8–9 and equal downhill recoveries; 20 min at RPE 6	rest	45 min at RPE 6	2 hr walk
off road; 3 miles (4.8 km)	rest	45 min at RPE 6–7	7 1/2 miles (12 km)
cross train 30–60 min	rest	45 min at RPE 6–7	8 1/2 miles (13.5 km)
cross train 30–60 min	rest	45 min at RPE 6–7	3 hr walk
off road; 3 1/2 miles (5.6 km)	rest	1 hr at RPE 6	10 miles (16 km)
10 min at RPE 5–6; 30 min incline at RPE 8; 10 min at RPE 5–6	rest	cross train 30–60 min	3 1/2 hr walk

running or walking?

If you can't find a walking marathon, see whether any of the running marathons have a walking event going on at the same time—many now do.

HOW LONG WILL IT TAKE?

A marathon provides 26 miles (41.8 km) of pleasure. If you are hoping for a good time but your main aim is to finish, use the time trial or a previous 6-mile (9.6-km) event or half-marathon to predict your finish time. You should add on another 5–10 percent of the overall time to allow for drink stops, a slower walking pace as you tire, or crowds and bottlenecks.

MPH	6 MILES [9.6km]	1/2-MARATHON	MARATHON
3	2 hr	4 hr 22 min	8 hr 45 min
3 1/4	1 hr 51 min	3 hr 55 min	7 hr 50 min
3 1/2	1 hr 43 min	3 hr 50 min	7 hr 40 min
3 3/4	1hr 36 min	3 hr 29 min	7 hr
4	1 hr 30 min	3 hr 16 min	6 hr 32 min
4 1/4	1 hr 25 min	3 hr 3 min	6 hr 6 min
4 1/2	1 hr 20 min	2 hr 50 min	5 hr 40 min
5	1 hr 12 min	2 hr 37 min	5 hr 14 min

◄◄ how's it going?

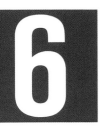

marathon walk continued

You may want to finish the event in a respectable time, but be realistic if this is your first race. You do not need to add anything on to the guidelines on the previous page because you will be aiming for a constant pace. Also, remember to pick up water as you are walking.

week 12— how's it going?

The 12th week is the week before your longest walk. Your walking time needs to total about 5½ hours, in which time you should aim to cover 20–22 miles (32–35.4 km) rather than doing the whole 26 miles (42 km). This training is followed by a two-week rest-and-taper period in which you reduce your training by up to 75 percent and increase your intake of carbohydrates to store glycogen. Remember to pay attention to any aches and pains—even at this stage, you should not ignore them. If your feet are aching from the long distances, cool buckets of water after a walk can be the ideal restorative.

WEEK	MONDAY	TUESDAY		
9	50 min at RPE 6–7	15 min at RPE 6–7; 4 x 4 min at RPE 8–9 with 2 min recoveries at RPE 4–5; 15 min at RPE 6–7		
10	55 min at RPE 6–7	10 min at RPE 6–7; 4 x 6 min at RPE 8–9 with 4 min recoveries at RPE 4–5; 10 min at RPE 6–7		
11	1 hr at RPE 6–7	10 min at RPE 6–7; 2, 4, 2, 6, 2, 4, 2 min at RPE 8–9 with half as long recoveries at RPE 4–5; 10 min at RPE 6–7		
12	1 hr at RPE 6–7	15 min at RPE 6–7; 10 x 2 min at RPE 8–9 with 2 min recoveries at RPE 4–5; 15 min at RPE 6–7		
13	1 hr at RPE 6–7	10 min at RPE 6–7; 4 x 4 min at RPE 8–9 with 2 min recoveries at RPE 4–5; 10 min at RPE 6–7		
14	30 min at RPE 6–7	15 min at RPE 6–7; 6 x 2 min at RPE 8–9 with 2 min recoveries at RPE 4–5; 15 min at RPE 6–7		
15	rest	10 min at RPE 6–7; 12, 6, 12 min at RPE 8–9 with 4 min recoveries at RPE 4–5; 15 min at RPE 6–7		
16	1 hr at RPE 6–7	rest		

event walking

Lifting one foot before the other one has landed is not allowed for a walking event, with disqualification the result. Be cautious and slow down if you are getting carried away. Better to be slow and finish than try to be too fast and end up barred from continuing. Always consider postponing the event if you are ill or injured. Don't try to push yourself through the pain barrier—the next event is never far away.

WEDNESDAY	THURSDAY	FRIDAY	SATURDAY	SUNDAY
3^1/$_2$ miles (5.6 km) at RPE 7–8	20 min at RPE 6; 6 x 2 min steep hill climb at RPE 8–9 and equal downhill recoveries; 20 min at RPE 6	rest	1 hr at RPE 6	12 miles (19 km)
4 miles (6.5 km) at RPE 6–7	off road; 4 miles (6.5 km)	rest	1 hr at RPE 6–7	14 miles (22.5 km)
4 miles (6.5 km) at RPE 7–8	cross train 30–60 min	rest	1 hr at RPE 6–7	4 hr walk
4^1/$_2$ miles (7 km) at RPE 6–7	off road; 4 miles (6.5 km)	rest	1 hr at RPE 5–6	16 miles (25.5 km)

◀◀ how's it going?

WEDNESDAY	THURSDAY	FRIDAY	SATURDAY	SUNDAY
5 miles (8 km) at RPE 6–7	cross train 30–60 min	rest	1 hr at RPE 5	18 miles (29 km)
3^1/$_2$ miles (5.5 km) at RPE 7–8	10 min at RPE 6; 8 x 2 min steep hill climb at RPE 8–9 and equal downhill recoveries; 10 min at RPE 6	rest	1 hr at RPE 5–6	20 miles (32 km) (final long walk)
3 miles (4.8 km) at RPE 6–7	cross train 30–60 min	rest	1 hr at RPE 7	8 miles (13 km)
1 hr at RPE 6–7	rest	1 hr at RPE 6–7	rest	**marathon**

6 advanced level weeklong trek

WEEK	MONDAY	TUESDAY	WEDNESDAY
1	rest	15 min at RPE 6–7; 2 x 4 min at RPE 8–9 with 2 min recoveries at RPE 4–5; 15 min at RPE 6–7	4 miles (6.5 km) at RPE 6–7 split into 2 sessions
2	rest	15 min at RPE 6–7; 2 x 6 min at RPE 8–9 with 4 min recoveries at RPE 4–5; 15 min at RPE 6–7	4 miles (6.5 km) at RPE 7–8 split into 2 sessions
3	rest	15 min at RPE 6–7; 4, 6, 4 min at RPE 8–9 with 4 min recoveries at RPE 4–5; 15 min at RPE 6–7	5 miles (8 km) at RPE 6–7 split into 2 sessions
4	rest	15 min at RPE 6–7; 6 x 2 min at RPE 8–9 with 2 min recoveries at RPE 4–5; 15 min at RPE 6–7	5 miles (8 km) at RPE 7–8 split into 2 sessions
5	rest	15 min at RPE 6–7; 3 x 4 min at RPE 8–9 with 2 min recoveries at RPE 4–5; 15 min at RPE 6–7	6 miles (9.6 km) at RPE 6–7 split into 2 sessions
6	rest	10 min at RPE 6–7; 3 x 6 min at RPE 8–9 with 4 min recoveries at RPE 4–5; 10 min at RPE 6–7	6 miles (9.6 km) at RPE 7–8 split into 2 sessions
7	rest	10 min at RPE 6–7; 6, 4, 2, 4, 6 min at RPE 8–9 with half as long recoveries at RPE 4–5; 10 min at RPE 6–7	6 miles (9.6 km) at RPE 7–8 split into 2 sessions
8	rest	15 min at RPE 6–7; 8 x 2 min at RPE 8–9 with 2 min recoveries at RPE 4–5; 15 min at RPE 6–7	7 miles (11 km) at RPE 6–7 split into 2 sessions

extreme climates

If you plan to go to a high, cold, hot, or humid place with a different climate to where you have been training, you should also take account of the different food and fluid requirements. If, for example, you are traveling in hot areas or at high altitudes, then eat more and stay well hydrated. Do not rely on local supplies of any essential food and equipment in far-off places, but rather take as much dried foods and bottled water as you need. Take tablets for unreliable water supplies, and research as much as you can about the region to prepare yourself before you travel.

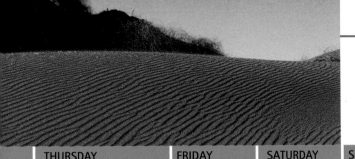

THURSDAY	FRIDAY	SATURDAY	SUNDAY
off road over different terrains; 2¹/₂ miles (4km)	1 hr at RPE 6–7 or rest	45 min at RPE 5–6	4 miles (6.5 km)
20 min at RPE 5–6; 15 min inclines at RPE 7–8; 20 min at RPE 5–6	1 hr at RPE 6–7 or rest	cross train 30–60 min	5 miles (8 km)
20 min at RPE 6; 8 x 1 min steep hill climb at RPE 8–9 and equal downhill recoveries; 20 min at RPE 6	1 hr at RPE 6–7 or rest	45 min at RPE 6	1 hr walk
off road over different terrains; 3 miles (4.8 km)	1 hr 10 min at RPE 6–7 or rest	45 min at RPE 6–7	6 miles (9.6 km)
cross train 1 hr	1 hr 20 min at RPE 6–7	45 min at RPE 6–7	7 miles (11 km)
off road over different terrains; 4 miles (6.5 km)	1¹/₂ hr at RPE 6–7 or rest	1 hr at RPE 6–7	2 hr walk
off road over different terrains; 5 miles (8 km)	1¹/₂ hr at RPE 6–7 (can split into 2 sessions)	1¹/₂ hr at RPE 6	9 miles (14.5 km)
30 min at RPE 5–6; 30 min inclines at RPE 8; 30 min at RPE 5–6	1¹/₂ hr at RPE 6–7 (can split into 2 sessions)	cross train 30–60 min	2 hr walk

week 6— how's it going?

If you are going on a trip with a group, make sure that you will not be holding them back. However, if you have followed this schedule you will be one of the fittest of the participants. As long as you stick to the schedule, there should be no concerns about your capability or fitness—just make sure that you stay injury-free.

6 weeklong trek continued

WEEK	MONDAY	TUESDAY	WEDNESDAY
9	rest	15 min at RPE 6–7; 4 x 4 min at RPE 8–9 with 2 min recoveries at RPE 4–5; 15 min at RPE 6–7	7 miles (11 km) at RPE 7–8 split into 2 sessions
10	rest	10 min at RPE 6–7; 4 x 6 min at RPE 8–9 with 4 min recoveries at RPE 4–5; 10 min at RPE 6–7	8 miles (13 km) at RPE 6–7 split into 2 sessions
11	rest	10 min at RPE 6–7; 2, 4, 2, 6, 2, 4, 2 min at RPE 8–9 with half as long recoveries at RPE 4–5; 10 min at RPE 6–7	8 miles (13 km) at RPE 7–8 split into 2 sessions
12	rest	15 min at RPE 6–7; 10 x 2 min at RPE 8–9 with 2 min recoveries at RPE 4–5; 15 min at RPE 6–7	9 miles (14.5 km) at RPE 6–7 split into 2 sessions
13	rest	10 min at RPE 6–7; 4 x 4 min at RPE 8–9 with 2 min recoveries at RPE 4–5; 10 min at RPE 6–7	10 miles (16 km) at RPE 6–7 split into 2 sessions
14	rest	15 min at RPE 6–7; 6 x 2 min at RPE 8–9 with 2 min recoveries at RPE 4–5; 15 min at RPE 6–7	11 miles (17.5 km) at RPE 7 split into 2 sessions
15	rest	10 min at RPE 6–7; 12, 6, 12 min at RPE 8–9 with 4 min recoveries at RPE 4–5; 15 min at RPE 6–7	12 miles (19 km) at RPE 6–7 split into 2 sessions
16	1 hr at RPE 7	rest	1 1/2 miles (2.5 km) at RPE 7

walking at altitude

Acute mountain sickness (AMS) can be a danger if you are walking at high altitude. Your body can acclimatize to reduced oxygen levels, but do not climb too quickly too soon. Symptoms of AMS include shortness of breath, headaches, and dizziness. Descending should clear a mild case: if it doesn't, seek medical attention. Also seek specialist advice on equipment, health, safety, and emergency procedures before setting out.

THURSDAY	FRIDAY	SATURDAY	SUNDAY
20 min at RPE 6; 6 x 2 min steep hill climb at RPE 8–9 and equal downhill recoveries; 20 min at RPE 6	1 hr 40 min at RPE 6–7 (can split into 2 sessions)	2 hr at RPE 6	11 miles (17.5 km)
off road over different terrains; 6 miles (9.5 km)	1 hr 50 min at RPE 6–7 (can split into 2 sessions) or rest	2 1/2 hr at RPE 6–7	11 1/2 miles (18.5 km)
off road over different terrains; 7 miles (11 km)	2 hr at RPE 6–7 (can split into 2 sessions)	2 hr 40 min at RPE 6–7	3 hr walk
30 min at RPE 6–7; 1 hr inclines at RPE 8; 30 min at RPE 6–7	2 1/2 hr at RPE 6–7 (can split into 2 sessions)	3 hr min at RPE 5–8	12 miles (19 km)
cross train 30–60 min	3 hr at RPE 6–7 (can split into 2 sessions)	3 hr at RPE 5–8	14 miles (22.5 km)
20 min at RPE 6; 8 x 2 min steep hill climb at RPE 8–9 and equal downhill recoveries; 20 min at RPE 6	3 hr at RPE 6–7 (can split into 2 sessions)	3 hr at RPE 6–8	6 hr walk
off road over different terrains; 8 miles (13 km)	4 hr at RPE 6–7 (can split into 2 sessions)	4 hr at RPE 6–7	4 hr walk
rest	2 hr at RPE 6–7 (can split into 2 sessions)	rest	beginning of walking vacation

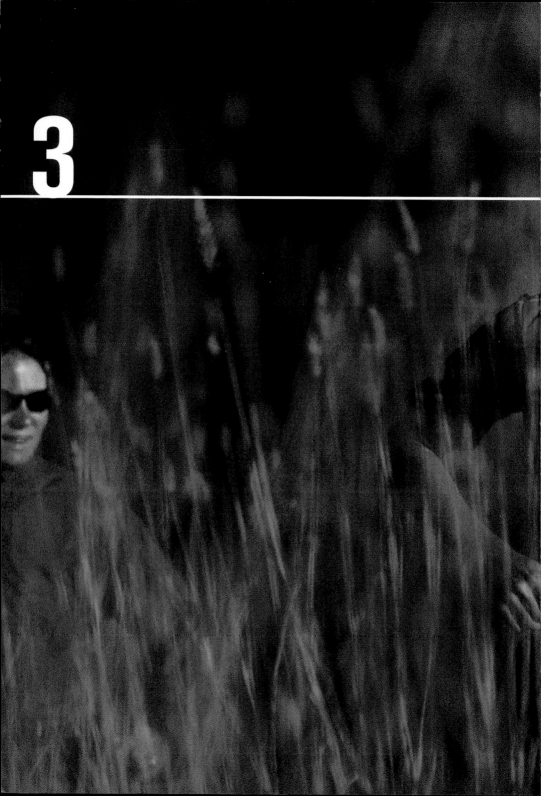

3

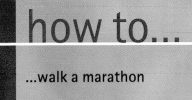

how to...

...walk a marathon

...walk lighter

...walk into long-term fitness

...walk a marathon

A marathon is a hard endurance test and should not be undertaken lightly, which is why it is so exhilarating to complete. You have trained hard, so you will be exhausted, stiff (no matter how fit you are), and there will have been moments when you have wondered why you are doing it at all. Yet the months of training will pale into insignificance when you cross the finish line. The audience support along the route keeps your spirits up, but it is your spirit and determination that will keep you going until the end. The key pointers to a successful event are listed below.

1 schedule in your walks

When you want to walk this sort of distance, you cannot afford to be sporadic in your training. Follow the marathon schedules, and build up to the marathon program. If your work schedule is hectic or other life events make the longer walks difficult, adapt the program or move your goal. It is easier and safer if you keep as close as possible to the schedule.

2 build up speed

Walking fast at least twice a week will build up your strength and speed for a marathon. It will also help your form and give new interest to the longer walks.

3 increase your walking time

It is not possible to train the body to walk for hours during an event without spending hours at a time training. Build up your times gradually, and try to walk on different surfaces to reduce soreness.

4 take time out

Training can take over your life. The desire to get faster and fitter can make rest seem like an unnecessary luxury. Don't fall into this trap—rest is a crucial part of the program, so follow the schedule.

preparation week

1 Walk at a leisurely pace over the first 5 days for no more than 20 minutes. Rest completely for the last 2 days.

2 Eat normally—this allows your body to build up its glycogen stores naturally alongside the reduction in your walking times.

3 Drink plenty, especially in the last few days.

4 Plan your travel arrangements. Arrange for friends and family to come and support you.

5 Do not forget warm clothes for the finish. Pack all you may need in your bag: you will be able to leave it with friends or with the event organizers.

6 Do not be tempted to take part if you are ill or recovering from illness. There is always another event.

7 Change nothing. New clothes, shoes, or food should wait until after the event. You know what works, so never change a winning formula.

the big day

1 Do not miss breakfast, and eat about 2 hours before the start. A small snack will help if the meal was a long time before.

2 Once you have started, stick with the main crowd until it thins out naturally. Pushing past other walkers in the early stages will only irritate you (and them) and delay your natural pace and technique.

3 Walk at least the first half of the distance at a comfortable pace. When you have passed the 18-mile (29-km) mark, pick up the pace a bit if your legs feel fine.

4 Drink small amounts frequently. Remember that thirst is a sign of dehydration. Regular sips also mean that you are less likely to need to stop to use the lavatory, although facilities will always be provided on the route.

5 Vary your pace throughout the walk, either to walk with others or simply to introduce some variety. For example, choose a slower pace while you drink or eat and a faster pace when you are heading toward a marker.

6 Eat at least 100 calories for each hour of walking to keep up your energy. Use quickly digested foods that you know are easy on your stomach.

7 Revel in your achievement as you go past the cheering crowds—you deserve it.

...walk lighter

(see pp. 31–32)

balance your health

Neither exercise nor calorie control alone is the answer to permanent weight management; it is important both to eat and to exercise regularly. Weight management is simply the result of matching your calorie needs to your calorie intake. Exercise should not just be seen as an excuse to eat more or as something to be omitted if you eat less, because many of the health benefits you get through exercising cannot be gained in any other way.

Effective weight-loss diets are only successful because they cut the calories down. Whether the diet involves cutting out an entire food group (see pp. 31–32) or using dietary aids, meaning low-calorie foods such as celery and carrots and other vegetables, the hard truth is that fad diets can never replace a normal, healthy eating pattern.

Putting on weight takes time. An almost invisible weight gain of just 1 lb (0.5 kg) a year adds up to an extra 20 lb (9 kg) in 20 years. Even maintaining your current weight and not gaining any more each year is good.

When you decide that you want to lose weight, no amount of knowledge about calories and food types or exercise regimens is going to work if your behavior is in conflict with these principles.

are your expectations realistic?

a Do you have a wardrobe full of clothes that you are keeping for when you lose weight?	**c** Have you been trying to lose weight for more than 2 years?
b Are you putting off doing something until you lose weight?	**d** Do you buy every new diet book hoping for the magic formula that will work for you?

If the answer to any of these questions is "yes," then write an honest list (you don't have to show it to anyone) of all the reasons that you want to lose weight. Then choose the three most compelling reasons and pin them in the places that you will look at frequently, such as on the bedroom mirror or on the refrigerator door (you can always write them in code if you don't want others to see them).

identify your weaknesses

Concentrate your efforts on changing your behavior whenever you answer "yes" to any of the following questions:

a Do you eat when you are bored?	**d** Do you put off your daily exercise until later that day, or at another time when you have more energy, the weather improves, or your friend will join you?
b Do you cook for a family and eat the leftovers?	
c Do you judge your appetite by the plate size?	**e** Do you lose your resolve when the scales don't reward you with a hard-earned reduction?

... walk into long-term fitness

Walking could be the one activity that keeps you fit and independent when other pursuits have lost their appeal. Stay strong and healthy with these simple tips for a long, satisfying walking routine.

make it your call
The pace and type of walk you choose may vary over time. Make sure your decision on how fast or how far you go is based on your fitness, rather than someone else's.

don't let the grass grow
Always keep moving, even if long walks are difficult. If you can't walk, try alternative activities, swimming, or armchair exercises—anything that keeps the muscles strong and the joints mobile.

walk your worries away
When the going gets tough, the tough get walking. You can't guarantee a stress-free life but you can make sure that you are fit enough to cope with any challenge that comes your way.

give it back
All the experience and enjoyment that you have gained can be used to help with local walks, events, or clubs. Your knowledge and attitude are valuable: you will feel it when your positive attitude influences others.

inspire and be inspired
There are so many benefits from walking that you would be selfish not to share them with others. Decide to try to introduce some new people to walking.

keep exploring on foot
Walk anywhere and everywhere—try new routes and rediscover old ones.

offer mutual support
The best motivation comes from family and friends. If you can motivate them to be active too, then there is no way you can lose.

get away
Make one of your annual breaks a walking holiday. See exotic or local places through new eyes as you take in the scenery at a walking pace.

index

acknowledgments

Special thanks to the YHA Adventure Shop for providing equipment; many thanks also to Sweatshop for kindly providing clothing and equipment.

Thanks also to the model Katy Bartlett .

Additional photography: Mike Good

Every effort has been made to credit everybody who appears in this book, and we apologize in advance for any unintentional omissions. We would be pleased to insert the appropriate acknowledgment in any subsequent edition of this publication.